Culture of Accidents

Michael Witmore

Culture of Accidents

Unexpected Knowledges in Early Modern England

Stanford University Press
Stanford, California 2001

Stanford University Press
Stanford, California

Printed in the United States of America

Library of Congress Cataloging-in-Publication Data

Witmore, Michael
Culture of accidents : unexpected knowledges in early modern England / Michael Witmore.
p. cm.
Includes bibliographical references and index.
ISBN 0-8047-3556-5 (cloth : alk. paper)
1. Accidents—History. 2. Philosophy, English. I. Title.

BD701.W44 2001
111'1—dc21 2001040028
CIP

This book is printed on acid-free, archival quality paper.

Original printing 2001
Last figure below indicates year of this printing:
10 09 08 07 06 05 04 03 02 01

Typeset at Stanford University Press in 10/13 Palatino

Acknowledgments

The ideas in this book were nourished by conversations that took place over the course of several years in Berkeley, San Francisco, Berlin, Los Angeles and Pittsburgh. The list of my interlocutors is a long one. To Amir Alexander, Emma Bianchi, Rachel Crawford, Dallas Denery, Barbara Donagan, Richard Doyle, Peter Gordon, Daniel Gross, Félipe Gutterriez, Carol Hamilton, Evelyn Fox Keller, Homay King, Jon Klancher, Jeffrey Knapp, Peggy Knapp, Jael Lehmann, Isaac Miller, Gregory Moynahan, Kellie Robertson, Scott Sandage, Randolph Starn, Banu Subramanium, John Tinkler and David Wittenberg, I am grateful for the opportunity to share these ideas and—through the detour of discussion—discover them anew.

While a graduate student at Berkeley, I benefited from the guidance of Stephen Greenblatt, who seemed never to fear the deep waters of Scholasticism into which I was venturing and was trusting enough not to dissuade me from writing about *Hamlet*. Barbara Shapiro introduced me to English natural philosophy and, with typical foresight, recognized that my initial interest in accidents was about to develop into a dissertation. During his final years at Berkeley, Amos Funkenstein convinced me that any study of early modern accidents would require a medieval prologue. Having taken his advice, I wish I could now share with him the results. Finally, Hayden White and Lorraine Daston (in Berlin) were generous with their opinions as the project evolved, looking over my shoulder from time to time as I put the pieces together.

Several institutions provided fellowship support, a place to work, and that thing called community without which it is difficult to think and write. I want to acknowledge the Department of Rhetoric and the Townsend Center for the Humanities at Berkeley, the Huntington Library in San Marino, the Max Planck Institute für Wissenschaftsgeschichte in Berlin, the Center for Medieval and Renaissance Studies at UCLA and the Department of English at Carnegie Mellon for their support while I was researching, writing and revising. I should not leave out my students in this list of debts, since they were the mostly willing test subjects for the analyses and readings that follow. I also want to thank three readers at Stanford University Press who provided feedback on the manuscript in its early stages. This advice led to substantial revisions of the first three chapters.

My friends and colleagues in Pittsburgh came to my rescue while I was finishing the book, assisting me through several months of recovery from a serious auto accident. The irony of this turn of events astounds me, but not the warmth and generosity of those who came to my aid. On this account I owe special thanks to Carol Hamilton, Barbara Johnstone, Kathy Newman and Scott Sandage for helping me to defy the restrictions of life with casts on hand and foot. John Bernstein and Peter Kavic provided research assistance in Pittsburgh and the editorial staff at Stanford University Press worked to remove the errors that were and are mine alone. I also want to thank Pamela Jackson for her keen readings of the manuscript as it evolved. Without her intellectual presence and adventurous spirit, the labor of writing would have overwhelmed the love. Finally, I want to thank my parents, who have always matched their support for my work with a ready interest in what it is about. This book is dedicated to them.

M.W.

Contents

Note on Modernization

When quoting early modern editions of texts in English, I have supplied the modern typographical equivalents of certain letters (*v, vv, u* and *ſ*). Titles of early modern editions have been shortened in the bibliography but are reproduced liberally in the notes. For the sake of consistency, titles, punctuation and publishing information for these works have all been keyed to the second edition of Pollard's and Redgrave's *Short-Title Catalogue of Books Printed in England, Scotland and Ireland, 1475–1640.*

Let us dismiss the accidental; for we have sufficiently determined its nature.

—Aristotle, *Metaphysics* 1027b

Introduction: A Narrative Wonder

Over the last two decades, wonder and wonders have come to occupy a special place in early modern studies. Under this rubric, an astonishing range of subjects has been assembled for analysis, topics as disparate as the early modern fascination with "curiosities," debates about the significance of monstrous births and prodigies, representations of the "marvels" of the New World and changes in the nature of philosophical curiosity.[1] This work has made clear the degree to which experiences of the singular, astonishing and unexpected captivated the early modern imagination, engaging both a poetic appetite for the "strange" and a philosophical curiosity about the causes of singular phenomena. Having located wonder somewhere in the fertile zone between knowing and feeling, scholars now have a more integrated story to tell about the interlocking realms of early modern poetics, politics and epistemology, one that foregrounds the relationship between the representational practices that produced wonder and the various early modern interests—philosophical, religious, and political—which those practices engaged.[2] As this story gets told in richer detail, we recognize that the early modern fascination with things strange and unexpected cuts a broad path across English intellectual and cultural life, linking the rise of an experimental science with the theological interest in portentous events, connecting the marvels of the stage with a self-conscious theatricalization of experience in politics and religious life.[3]

Given the widespread interest in wonder, it is surprising that one of its most traditional sources—accidental events—has gone largely unstudied.[4] Accidents are some of the most luminous and enigmatic events to be found in early modern texts, appearing regularly on stage, in popular news reports, in theological texts and in philosophical treatises. Whenever they occur, accidents have the power to startle and amaze, inviting individuals to reflect on the causes and meaning of events that defy the human capacity for prudence, calculation and knowledge. This affective state or "passion" had already been linked to accidental events in the tradition of Aristotelian poetics, a tradition that was being revived in the sixteenth century as the *Poetics* became available to European readers.[5] Accidents, Aristotle writes in this text, are particularly qualified to provoke wonder in the theatrical spectator when they mix the spontaneous with the purposeful in suggestive ways. Such events are most marvelous because they have the appearance of design in them, he points out, and a plot that employs this device of the meaningful accident or chance event is "necessarily finer" than others.[6]

This glowing recommendation was not lost on early modern playwrights who packed their plays with "casualties," "mishaps," and "sudden accidents." But while accidents made for good drama—Jonson, Webster and Shakespeare regularly made use of them on stage—they presented a challenge to both the theology of the Reformation and the long-standing philosophical tradition of Aristotelian metaphysics. On the one hand, the early modern belief in "special providence" dictated that all events, no matter how unexpected or inconsequential, are actively brought about by a "disposing" God. Strictly speaking, there are no accidents in a providential world, something that early modern theologians such as John Calvin and his English interpreters were quick to point out.[7] As Calvin wrote in his landmark *Institutes of the Christian Religion*, "[T]he providence of God, as it is taught in Scripture, is opposed to fortune and fortuitous accidents," a dictum which suggested that the very idea of accidents was a theological absurdity.[8] On the other hand, accidents had for centuries been excluded as an object of knowledge in Aristotelian metaphysics, itself still a powerful intellectual force in the seventeenth century. According to Aristotle and his Scholastic interpreters, there could be no science of accidents; by definition these events had unique causes rather than general ones and so could not be brought into the purview of genuine philosophical inquiry.[9]

Given the reluctance of writers like Calvin and Aristotle to admit accidents as either a category of analysis or an object of knowledge, it is tempting to assume that early modern accidents were either impossible (because of God's providence) or unknowable (because they had no regular, general causes). Just the opposite is the case, however. Even a casual survey of early modern texts turns up repeated declarations that certain events come to pass "by accident," even if such events are really a more subtle form of divine action. Indeed, "accidents"—sudden, lamentable, happy, doleful, wonderful—occur in abundance during the period and are regularly described as such. They are even divided into a number of recognizable types. The unexpected meeting in the marketplace, the chance encounter with pirates or robbers, the hair's-breadth deliverance from danger or sudden death by a falling object: events like these were the common stock of the early modern imagination, easily recognizable as the kind of thing that happens once in a while. And while the word "accident" had the generic meaning of "event" during the sixteenth and seventeenth centuries, it nevertheless bore long-standing associations with the operations of chance and Fortune, those inscrutable pagan agencies that Christian writers like Calvin were working so hard to dismiss or refashion. Just as important, the word "accident" resonated with an immense body of learned thought on the nature of these events, associations that we can trace even into some of the least "intellectual" texts of the period.

Within natural philosophy, moreover, the accident would become increasingly significant as techniques for acquiring knowledge about nature began to change. Unlike the physics and metaphysics of the Scholastics, the natural philosophy that took shape in the seventeenth-century writings of Francis Bacon emphasized the need for "experiment" in the pursuit of knowledge.[10] The "contrived event" of the experiment, as Peter Dear has called it, might at first seem at odds with the spontaneous character of an accident.[11] Bacon, however, identified a fundamental similarity between both occurrences: accidents and experiments require an unusual disposition of circumstances, which is what makes both a powerful engine for discovery. Bacon's equation of experiment with accident—and here I am broaching one of the major claims of the book—marked an end to the accident's long-standing marginalization within philosophy; it also expressed a more widespread appreciation for the ways in which such spontaneous events were nevertheless somehow "contrived." Accidents were, in fact, a model for a certain kind of indirect action, a spontaneous form of revelation traditionally associated with the female goddess Fortuna, whom Bacon wanted to imitate in a regime of deliberate experimentation. Accidents also represented an instance of deviation in the usual course of things; their power to distract or estrange onlookers from habitual patterns of expectation and attention thus gave them unusual epistemological force in the skeptical context of the seventeenth century.[12]

Rather than sitting at the margins of intellectual and cultural life, then, accidents—like other marvels and wonders—captivated the early modern imagination and patterned some of its most distinctive modes of interpretation. This book is an attempt to describe some of these modes, showing how a mixture of intellectual distinctions and problems developed in the Aristotelian philosophical tradition were diffused across a truly astonishing range of early modern texts, some of them quite well known, others which are rarely read. In part, this is the story of how an abstraction moved out of the fertile pastures of Scholastic philosophy to acquire a cultural life of its own in the decades surrounding the turn of the seventeenth century. To the extent that it charts the development of a canonical concept within Scholasticism and its circulation through several early modern discursive domains—Shakespearean drama, Baconian natural philosophy, early modern theologies of providence, and a genre of popular wonder literature that chronicled "accidents"—this volume is a genealogy of an idea, or in the more traditional sense, an intellectual history.[13]

But the intellectual ferment over these events must itself be understood as part of a larger cultural engagement with accidents in the early modern period, one that a strictly philosophical analysis can only hint at. For early modern accidents are not simply a type of event with curious philosophical consequences; they are a regular feature of stories and storytelling, which means that their significance extends beyond the province of metaphysical reflection into other areas where narrative is a conduit for knowledge and experience. In addition to serving as a lightning rod for debates about God's providence, for example, we find the accident at the center of Shakespeare's highly reflexive theatrical practice, engaging basic questions about the nature of theatrical artifice and the relationship between the playwright's ordered world and that of a providential God. The prevalence of that analogy between world and stage, itself a staple of royal political rhetoric and post-Reformation theology, also meant that the accident was capable of generating powerful ideological effects, transforming the world of lived experience into a fiction whose narrative devices and conventions seemed scripted by an all-powerful being.[14] When we examine some of these effects in popular religious literature about "accidents," we find that accidents have a rhetoric and poetics of their own, one that binds their ideological force to certain genres of fiction and, in the case of Bacon, certain gendered notions of discovery and action. Finally, we see that as accidents become associated with theatrical display, they are increasingly viewed as a source of knowledge. This view of accident as an opportunity for revelation in the broadest sense depends, I will argue, on its association with narrative "contriving," an artificial quality that links the accident quite literally with the notion of "experiment" as it emerges in Francis Bacon's natural philosophy.

Words such as "narrative," "knowledge," and "revelation" should begin to suggest the cultural-epistemological thrust of the analyses that follow. On the one hand, this book charts an intellectual shift that saw accidents transformed from an epistemological dead end into a source of knowledge in the early modern period, whether that knowledge was of God, nature, or the hidden plots of individuals. On the other, it identifies some of the representational strategies that enhanced the accident's association with revelation and knowledge, particularly those that placed accidents in a theatrical frame, thereby cementing their association with contrivance and status as a narrative device. As I will argue in the chapters that follow, these two developments are related, which is why I have regularly tried to bring accounts of the narrative practices at work in early modern texts into contact with the intellectual currents they engaged. This approach of merging the intellectual and cultural is not arbitrary, but a consequence of the curious status that the accident has in early modern texts, both as an object of knowledge and as a narrative device. Since these two features of the accident—what I call their "categorical instability" and their "rhetoricity"—are a recurring motif in the analyses that follow, I would like to introduce them at the outset before continuing with more focused discussion in individual chapters.

As a species of event, accidents are a kind of intellectual monstrosity—a mixture of fact and fiction, artifice and spontaneity, and ultimately, event and action. This categorical instability is crucial for their status as early modern wonders, which as a group tended to straddle important ontological divisions between the natural and the supernatural, the fictional and the real.[15] When, for example, Francis Bacon considered monstrous births in his philosophical writings, he compared these "wondrous" creations of nature to fantastic works of art. In an astonishing passage from Book Two of his *Advancement of Learning*, he suggests that, by studying "Heteroclites or Irregulars of Nature," we can discover the techniques nature employs in crafting these most extravagant productions and eventually employ them ourselves.[16] Wonder cabinets, which enjoyed a huge popularity during the period, also blurred the boundaries of natural and artificial, gathering together exquisite examples of the "sports" or "jests" of nature, such as stones bearing patterns of clouds and trees, shells that seemed to have been shaped by a sculptor, or crystals with elaborate geometrical patterns.[17] The fact that many of these patterns could have been explained within the prevailing natural philosophy as the result of chance—as the "accidental" development of a significant pattern—only enhanced their paradoxical linkage with artistic creation.[18]

Like Bacon's monsters and the curious sports of nature, accidental events blended the properties of nature and art in highly suggestive ways. While these events were often understood to come about spontaneously, as a result of a rare concurrence of circumstances, they also fulfilled some recognizable purpose and so savored of artifice and premeditation. A falling object, for example, could kill someone who was unfortunate enough to be standing where it fell. Death in such cases could be explained entirely with reference to natural causes: heavy objects fall, the vital spirits are stilled by a sudden blow to the head. But if that person happened to be a murderer, the accident might seem to come about for a reason, perhaps as a kind of divine justice. Echoes of this example from Aristotle's *Poetics* can be found in a number of early modern texts, where death-by-falling-object is virtually a generic formula for divine punishment. The fact that such a formula could be deployed by a broad range of English writers suggests the degree to which two ontologically distinct realms—those of poesy and history, as Francis Bacon divided them—had a common boundary in accidental events. A whole range of early modern writers were drawn to the accident's curiously contrived qualities—some like Bacon for philosophical reasons, others like William Shakespeare because they posed fundamental questions about the nature of theatrical experience. Still other writers, providentialists such as William Gouge, John Field, and Phillip Stubbes, were attracted to the possibility that dramatic accidents happening in the world might persuade wayward individuals to renew their faith, subjecting them to a "buried" knowledge of God's power.

We ought to think of accidents as existing halfway between the realms of fact and fiction during this period, a quality that makes them appealing to a broad range of interests. This categorical instability allows accidents to serve as a passageway between realms of experience that are traditionally thought to exclude one another. When, for example, a person in the world is struck by a falling object and killed—and it happens often enough in the popular "accident" literature which chronicled the mishaps of wayward sinners—the individual who suffers the fatal blow becomes a protagonist in some earthly drama. It is this sense of drama that Calvin and other religious writers are keen to indulge when they recommend that individuals pay attention to accidents, "regarding" the daily examples of providential action in their immediate surroundings. Conversely, when accidents happen on stage, they import a material feature of the world—its blind bustle of things combining in unforeseen ways—into the thoroughly contrived space of art. Possessed of both the indifferent necessity of fact and the weird symmetry of fiction, accidents blurred the difference between real and imagined worlds, drawing one to the other without necessarily securing a boundary between the two.

This connection with fiction should be made more concrete, however, since the specific art associated with early modern accidents is that of the theater. Here we can appreciate more precisely how a widespread belief in providence affected the way in which accidents were represented by religious writers, philosophers and dramatists who placed them on public view. No doubt such a belief encouraged individuals to attend to unexpected events and, at times, anguish over their inscrutability. But providentialism did not wipe out accidents; rather, it fostered a culturewide enterprise of narrating these unexpected events with an eye toward their intrinsic drama and providential meaning.[19] Having a narrative framework in which to place these events was essential to recognizing them as accidents, and this necessary link between accident and narrative is something I will be returning to throughout this study. Here, however, I want to point out one of the ways in which the substantial cultural and narrative resources of early modern theatrical genres like tragedy were brought to bear on representations of accidents with profound ideological effects.

The theater was a ready model for an accident-prone world, supplying a controlled space in which to plot sudden events and reflect on their causes. Like accidents on stage, those in the world were subject to a curious form of premeditation: while they might appear to come about spontaneously, accidents were actually arranged by some kind of superordinant agency that staged them for a dramatic or didactic end. The world was a "theater of God's judgement," as Thomas Beard called it in his translation of a text by Jean de Chassanion, a fact which popular writers never tired of reminding their readers of, even if it might temporarily be forgotten.[20] In 1623, one anonymous writer characterized the situation as follows:

> [T]he world is a Theater, and the actions therof a continued Scene whereby our Lord hath manifested unto us these designes of his impartial judgments, the effects whereof he doth reveale, although the intention and purpose of them be kept secret unto himselfe.[21]

For this writer, the specific design or intention behind the theatrical scene of the world cannot be fathomed. The ultimate illegibility of the theatrical action presents no obstacle to the recognition of providence, however, since it is the quality of contrivance itself—what Calvin describes as God's ability to "dispose . . . al things in fittest opportunitie"—that makes the accident a conspicuous form of divine action.[22] Like the craft of "indirection" which is constantly being plied in Shakespeare's *Hamlet*, the craft of providential action is one of arranging circumstances and agents, of setting this particular character out on a meditative walk just as another is about to cross the path. Such encounters can be striking in the theater precisely because they unfold in a literal space: on the stage, being somewhere can be as much a cause of what happens as saying or doing something.

By linking the artifice of accidents to theatrical disposition, early modern writers created a powerful (because ontologically ambiguous) scheme with which to explore these events; the theatrical analogy had the potential to transform any spontaneous event into a fictional "device" or theatrical "conceit." If both the world and the stage were thoroughly contrived situations, subject to the disposing whims of a supervising author, then even the most apparently spontaneous event might be a more devious form of action. Here a basic philosophical and narrative distinction begins to dissolve around the accident, that between events (which simply happen of themselves) and actions (which are directed from without).[23] Because early modern accidents are regularly the objects of some more global "practice" or conceit—because they can be juggled by an agent whose craft and passion is that of arranging—they are always more than a mere occurrence but less than a deliberate "authorial" act.[24] In addition to straddling the boundaries between art and nature, life and fiction, then, accidents sit in a middle state of action during this period: no matter how spontaneous they seem, they bear the marks of a subtle, "dispositional" form of agency that is understood to organize theatrical action.

Such paradoxes thrilled the early modern writers examined in this study, inviting them to contemplate the convertible wonders of nature and art in the realm of narrative happenings. For readers and writers alike, accidents did in narrative terms what monsters and other marvels did to some basic ontological categories of physics and metaphysics: they combined them in a tantalizing mix, stoking curiosity and providing a glimpse into some hidden order that only a "contrived" event might reveal. The larger reason for examining this kind of categorical instability is not simply to identify a characteristic form of intellectual pleasure but also to relate this new intermediary quality of the accident to a specific epistemological habit of thought during this period: that of associating contrivance with discovery.[25] We find a powerful source for this association in the philosophy of Francis Bacon, who repeatedly argued that experiments were a deliberate means of arriving at hidden truths which were otherwise revealed only by accident. Bacon's views express a more pervasive shift toward a conception of nature in which the truth is hidden instead of conspicuous, a conception which in the past had been limited to an esoteric tradition of medieval secrets and arcana.[26] We can detect this tendency to think of the truth as hidden or buried in a range of early modern interests not specifically connected with natural philosophy; it is present in the culturewide obsession with uncovering hidden truths of infidelity, for example, or in the pervasive paranoia surrounding court politics—even in the studied ease of the courtier, hiding his well-rehearsed presentation in deliberately casual moments of *sprezzatura*. All of these impulses contribute to a sense that the true "craft" behind appearances is hidden and will remain so unless actively sought out and discovered.[27]

For many, the best way to discover such a hidden craft was to employ another. Thus, on the one hand, we find an experimental attitude developing that associates the artificial manipulation of experience with the uncovering of latent patterns of natural action. Regardless of how those manipulations are supposed to take place or the specific causes they are supposed to illuminate, the basic posture toward knowledge—thinking of it as an understanding of the hidden craft in either the natural world or that of human actions—is already well developed in the early decades of the seventeenth century.[28] The brand of "special providence" developed by Calvin and elaborated by his English interpreters is equally important for understanding this emergent habit of thought. Calvin and others repeatedly point out the way in which a latent knowledge of God's providential presence is uncovered in encounters with accidents. The simultaneous recognition and discovery of God's power follows, on this account, from an appreciation of the theatrical quality of these unexpected events; the spontaneous contrivance of the accident effectively transforms it into a conduit for knowledge of God's existence and power. For both the special providentialist and the experimentalist, then, knowing and contriving go hand in hand. The accidental event is a starting point for reflection in both cases, either on the power of God to control worldly events or the power of the individual to repeat such "accidents" in a deliberate program of experimentation.

As subsequent chapters demonstrate, the curious ontological status of the accident allowed it to become deeply entwined with early modern theatrical practice, providential ideology, and natural philosophy. But these events were also linked to the act of narrative representation, a process that enhanced the accident's spontaneous "purposiveness" by relating it to a communal set of interests. To the accident's categorical instability, then, we must now add another quality—rhetoricity—which enabled it to find a niche outside metaphysics in drama, popular marvel literature, natural philosophy and providential theology. Here we cease to think of accidents in epistemological terms, as spontaneously contrived events that disclose hidden forms of order, and instead begin to understand them as occasions for storytelling and the expression of immanent forms of value. That is the perspective which will allow us to discern a culture of accidents in the early modern period, rather than a "problem" or "idea."

The building block of accident narratives is the example, a compact descriptive sequence with a beginning, middle and end in which something happens to an intention, real or implied. For example, a man sets sail on a ship for one destination and is met unexpectedly by pirates who take him away to another. Both the man and his purpose here are forced to swerve when the pirates arrive; indeed, the example starts to become a story at the instant when an intention (embodied in the man's "course") becomes subject to alteration. Such examples of "intentions crossed" tend to migrate across different discursive domains, so we find the same accident type—someone's unexpectedly changing course in a journey after a meeting with pirates or a storm—as an illustration in a philosophical text (Aristotle's *Metaphysics*), as an example in a theological treatise (in Calvin's *Institutes*) and as a plot twist in a play (Shakespeare's *Hamlet*). The "accident" itself remains true to its conventional type, but its significance shifts depending upon the discursive domain in which it appears.[29]

While their forms are somewhat conventional, accidents must nevertheless possess certain narrative qualities if they are to be recognized as such. Recalling an earlier example, it is possible to record an accidental death as follows: a man is sitting, watching a public performance of some kind, when he is crushed by a heavy object. This is not much of a story, because it lacks important details. Who is the man and what is his history? Did anyone push the object that came hurtling down? When Aristotle uses the example in his description of an ideal tragic plot, he adds the following information: the man is the murderer of Mitys, the object that kills him has fallen spontaneously, that object is a statue of Mitys himself. Now the story has a narrative arc which can engage the spectator's sense of what is probable, meaningful, or deserving of praise or punishment. Would the accident seem as significant in a culture in which murder was not seen as a cause for revenge? Would the murderer's death, moreover, stand out as an ironic turn of events for spectators who did not believe in providence—for example, a group of Epicureans? The details that add drama are the same details that engage a communal (and so contingent) sense of right and wrong, likely and unlikely. The value of the accident to a plot depends, in other words, on the value of this outcome for a particular group of people.

Accidents thus do not simply happen in a cultural void, but result when certain narrative conventions (what we usually describe as plot) come into contact with communal beliefs about what is likely, valuable or purposive. This is tantamount to saying that the accident is a narrative artifact, one that draws its power to astonish from assumptions about what is usually the case and, more important, assumptions about the value of certain outcomes or events. We can get a better grasp on this process whereby rhetorical form and cultural assumptions collide to produce an accident in a more extended example, this time from London in the early seventeenth century. In the winter of 1623, a group of around three hundred Catholics and Protestants gathered in the top floor of a garret house in the Blackfriars district of London to hear a sermon by the Jesuit preacher Robert Drury. Packed into the third story of the building, the auditors were listening to the priest when the floor suddenly gave way and nearly one hundred people were instantly killed. The event was a citywide sensation, not only because so many perished in a single "downfall" but also because in James's Protestant England, Catholics appeared to be punished in the act of practicing their faith. All over London, individuals began to ask questions about this sudden interruption of a Catholic "vesper," one whose circumstances seemed the stuff of high tragedy. Were Catholics being punished for their beliefs, meeting their end in a grim "theater" of God's wrath? Were Protestants being asked to withhold their censure in a show of humility at the awful scene? The event seemed a virtual invitation to religious speculation, and a stream of narratives appeared soon after which provided different sectarian perspectives.

Like most accidents, the one that occurred in Blackfriars was capable of supporting a range of interpretations, few of which could be falsified or dismissed by the available evidence. The event was simultaneously dramatic and prosaic; even if it was unprecedented, it was not the stuff of miracles, which meant that its status as an accident or coincidence needed to be considered with special care. The pamphlets and broadsides that followed the event catered to widespread uncertainty about just how such an "accident" ought to be explained. Indeed, the printed accounts that followed the Blackfriars accident are really a case study in how accidents become a popular print phenomenon, "happening" again and again in the narratives which set them out for eager readers. (I discuss this particular case in detail later on in the book.) Several aspects of the Blackfriars accident and its aftermath are significant, given the rhetorical and cultural perspective outlined above. First, the sectarian differences that were expressed in descriptions of the event—and these differences surfaced immediately—were not just appended to an indifferent recounting of the accident, but shaped those accounts from the bottom up. One writer sympathetic to the Catholic cause, for example, compared the preacher's strange misgivings before entering the garret house to the portentous hesitations of Julius Caesar before going out to meet his death. The accident thus transforms an individual (here, the unfortunate Drury) into a protagonist in a dramatic scene, qualifying him for any number of stories which could be used to make sense of what happened from a particular interested perspective.

The question of perspective leads us to a more general paradox surrounding the identification of accidents in this or any other historical period. In order to recognize an event as an accident in the first place, one must already have placed that event into some larger, communal scheme of value. In fact, accidents are a prime occasion for the recognition and expression of communal values which shape narrative representations of "what happened." We can appreciate the significance of this point by examining an incidental detail about the Blackfriars accident that circulated among those who wrote about it. Thomas Goad, an eyewitness to the event, was competing with several other writers to produce the first printed account of it. Because Goad was also in the position of censor, he is thought to have delayed the publication of competing narratives, poaching details that he himself had not witnessed or heard. Goad's most interesting appropriation was a story about a young girl who looked at the ruined building and was said to have announced that this would "prove a great scandall to their religion."[30] Why was this detail so tantalizing? Because it proved to early modern readers that even a child, untutored in the ways of providence and only superficially aware of the sectarian conflicts of the age, could recognize the significance of the event. There was a deeper truth about the accident which the girl had spontaneously announced without necessarily grasping its significance: that the downfall happened for a reason and so had a value *for* some people, whether that value was positive or negative.

Even a child could recognize the providential purpose in the terrible accident. Goad had found a powerful story indeed, since the incident with the child made the recognition of providence a spontaneous, almost reflexive event rather than a deliberate, reasoned conclusion. But the child was really only doing what everyone else had to do in order to recognize the accident as such: she had to engage some communal sense of the reasons *for* which things happen and, from that sense, anticipate the value of the accident for a group of people. Without this immanent sense of value, the event would not even have qualified as an accident in the Aristotelian sense—a natural occurrence with no regular efficient cause. Rather, the "lamentable downfall" of this large group of people would be "something that happened," a bundle of rotten timber plunging downward with a heavy weight on top of it. The fact that no one was ready to describe the event in such commonplace terms (at least, no one was ready to do so in print) says a great deal about the readiness of the early modern mind to grasp providential purpose in any occasion.

One further point ought to be made about the process of recognition described above. The term "value" here does not refer simply to an instrumental purpose that might be grasped in accidental events. Rather, this properly cultural form of value encompasses both a hermeneutic meaning which the accident expresses and the goal or "end" which the event is understood to serve. The former, hermeneutic value, is a property of narrative, residing in the arrangement of agents that makes the accident possible. The latter purpose or "end," on the other hand, is the instrumental one—ascribed to some hypothetical doer who can be imagined to perform the accidental "deed." Only by including both aspects of the accident's value in our analysis, reflecting on its narrative meaning and the specific purposes which it was thought to accomplish, can we understand the diffuse teleological end "for which" an accident happens in this period. Indeed, what makes the accident a powerful focal point for cultural interest in this or any other historical period is the way in which it puts this plural sense of cultural value into play, allowing such value to be shifted, contested, or openly debated in either narrative or dialectical form. This contest can take the form of a debate over the accident's relation to known causes, in which case the debate is either practical or philosophical, or it can take the form of a reading of a particular accident in which some overarching meaning (and by extension, some source of meaning) is interpreted along poetic lines, often in the form of a concrete narrative.

What makes the accident particularly powerful in an early modern context, however, is the degree to which the fund of knowledge about the causes at work in the world and the nature of providential order was itself undergoing dramatic changes. In order to understand the broad significance of some of these shifts, we must take a longer philosophical view of the accident, trying to understand the conceptual problems it poses and the epistemological boundaries it marks out. The first two chapters of this book offer such an analysis, presenting the accident as an intellectual, rhetorical and theological *topos* for learned writers from Aristotle through the Scholastics and on to Jean Calvin, the sixteenth-century theologian who began to reverse the orthodox treatment of accidents by linking them to knowledge and revelation. After this extended introduction, I turn to specific early modern instances in which real or fictional accidents engaged some of the broader philosophical and cultural issues discussed above. Two chapters focus on plays by William Shakespeare, who perhaps more than any other early modern writer assayed the structural possibilities of the accident as a narrative device, turning it this way and that to discover its theatrical, affective, and even philosophical possibilities. Another chapter takes up the natural philosophy of Francis Bacon, whose program for philosophical reform suggested that accident and fortune might be imitated in the process of experimentation—a powerful reversal of the prevailing Aristotelian bias against these events. Finally, a chapter on the Blackfriars accident of 1623 explores how the theatrical and ideological force of this event could be opposed to (but also harmonized with) the naturalistic explanations that characterized learned discussion of marvelous events in the seventeenth century.

Each of the following chapters raises questions that resonate with a long-standing tradition of thinking about accidents as a "convergence" or "meeting" of independent lines of causation. While this orienting metaphor of crossing trajectories was not always explicit in early modern discussions of accidents, it was tacitly affirmed in narrative representations which made accidental meetings the turning point in spatial patterns of action; this was particularly true of the stage, where the spatial disposition of actors could itself become a significant means of advancing the plot. The pre-eminent source of this metaphor of convergence was Aristotle, who argued that certain events had no proper cause because they resulted from the accidental meeting of regularly acting efficient causes such as nature or the will.[31] By explaining accidents in terms of such meetings, Aristotle created an opportunity for subsequent writers to appropriate this metaphor for their own purposes. The questions which emerged in learned debates about accidents would ultimately revolve around the possibility that such meetings might themselves become an object of deliberate manipulation. Such questions, and the Aristotelian terms in which they were posed, are the subject of the next chapter.

CHAPTER 1

Early Modern Accidents and an Aristotelian Tradition

In the final scene of *Hamlet*, Horatio delivers the murderous events of Shakespeare's play to posterity in the language of accident, asking those who remain to let him:

> speak to th' yet unknowing world
> How these things came about. So shall you hear
> Of carnal, bloody, and unnatural acts,
> Of accidental judgements, casual slaughters,
> Of deaths put on by cunning and forced cause;
> And, in this upshot, purposes mistook
> Fallen on the inventors' heads.[1] (5.2.332–38)

Horatio knows that the story of what "came about" will be one in which deliberate actions are brutally severed from their expected results. Nature has been frustrated by unnatural acts, progress and plots defied by an indifference of the world to ready manipulation. The sense of causal disconnection and metaphysical drift that suffuses the play has finally, in this closing summary, found expression in a powerful cluster of adjectives: unnatural, accidental, and casual.

Of the three words used here, "accidental" has a special intellectual force in the early modern context: it is an Aristotelian diagnosis of events that defy human powers of calculation and foresight. Like arrows shot upward, "purposes" have been launched into the sky only to land on the "inventors' heads," a circular kind of disaster which parallels that which befalls the proverbial engineer who is "hoist with his own petard."[2] Following the diagnostic cue, spectators are led to consider the ironic force of errancy in the play, one which assures that various schemes and devices will not only stray or miscarry but also that they will return to do the "inventor" some harm.[3] Given the covert nature of the crimes that have been revealed here (beginning with the stealthy poisoning of King Hamlet), the conspicuous failure of plots on stage testifies to a diffuse brand of justice, ungraspable in its means but nevertheless obvious in its purpose.

The paradoxes surrounding this kind of accidental "purposiveness" had long been the province of philosophy, which may explain why Horatio would invoke that tradition at the conclusion of the play. But what exactly did the word "accident" mean to the audience listening to the scholar from Wittenberg's last words? How did this term from Aristotelian metaphysics help early modern spectators to grasp the larger poetic and religious significance of the accidents in Shakespeare's tragedy? Such questions quickly lead us from the play to the cultural moment in which it was performed. If we fix our attention on that moment, we find that Shakespeare and his turn-of-the-century audience share a common sensibility: both are fascinated with the power of accidental events to frustrate or complete human desires, to create spectacular moments of human drama, and perhaps most important, to reveal some underlying order that links the theatrical and created worlds.

Indeed, the semantic and philosophical resonances of "accident" during this period suggest that this closing scene of *Hamlet* taps into a widespread early modern interest in the unexpected and unforeseen, an interest that extends far beyond the appetite of Elizabethan and Jacobean playgoers for sudden dramatic turns of events on stage.[4] The word itself had a wide range of uses in the early modern lexicon. Lamentable "accidents" of fire, earthquake, flood or storm could befall any human enterprise. There were "accidents" of war, "accidental" meetings of friends, "accidental deliverances" from enemies and "accidental judgments" on sinners. Lovers, courtiers, and philosophers made sudden discoveries of infidelity, intrigue, or the secrets of nature on "accidental occasions." The "accidents of the times" could bode well or ill for a king surveying the historical physiognomy of his reign. When Shakespeare's audience heard Horatio's evocation of "accidental judgments and casual slaughters," it would have recognized several of the key events in the play—the meeting with pirates at sea, the *chaude melée* exchange of rapiers, the detour of the poisoned cup, perhaps even Hamlet's murder of Polonius—as being part of this broader category of accidental events.

The next two chapters offer an analytic account of that category, exploring first the contemporary meanings of the term Horatio uses and then situating these meanings within a learned tradition that assayed the accident's place in organized schemes of knowledge, causality and providential governance.[5] My initial move in this chapter on the Aristotelian genealogy of the "accident" will be to explore the semantic range of this word around the turn of the seventeenth century, a range of use which suggests that "accident" could refer to any noteworthy or astonishing event which had not been predicted in advance. This type of event was associated with at least two other traditions besides the philosophical one: that of Fortune and the romance on the one hand, and a rhetorical-legal tradition on the other. A brief examination of these other traditions below will suggest that both the law and the romance (with its local goddess *Fortuna*) tended to resolve the accident into either an action or an event, eliminating the amphibious quality of "spontaneous contrivance" that made accidents such a provocative object of philosophical analysis. Moving on to a discussion of Aristotle, we find that it is precisely this amphibious quality of accidents that comes into focus when he attempts to exclude them from his metaphysical scheme. In isolating an orphaned, hypothetical purpose that gets attached to accidental events, Aristotle provides us with a more precise understanding of the accident's value as a theatrical device and a narrative artifact, both of which emerge when the concept is subjected to analytic pressure.

Beginning with "Accidents"

One meaning of the term "accident" in the early modern period was generic, similar to the word "event" as it is used now. Modern use of the word "accident" elides this sense, for which the *Oxford English Dictionary* supplies the following definition: "an occurrence, incident, or event."[6] "Accident" is derived from the Latin verb *accidere* (to fall down), which was itself used in classical, medieval, and subsequent Latin texts with the sense of "to happen" or "to occur."[7] The earliest recorded use of the term in English appears to be circa 1374, in Chaucer's *Troilus and Creseyde*: "This accident so petous was to here." The word is still used in this way during the late sixteenth and early seventeenth centuries, as we can see from the titles of several books and broadsides.[8] One book published in 1601, for example, promises *A true report of all the proceedings of Grave Mauris before the towne of Bercke: with all the accidentes that happened in the besiedge of the same, since the 12. day of June last.* A similar generic sense for the word "accident" appears in the title of Edward Hake's, *Newes out of Powles Churchyarde now newly renued and amplifyed according to the accidents of the present time.*[9]

Many of these books qualify the word "accident" with adjectives such as "strange," "wonderful," and "memorable." In 1599, for example, we find a book entitled: *A strange and miraculous accident happened in the cittie of Purmerent, on New yeeres even last past 1599. Of a yong child which was heard to cry in the mothers wombe before it was borne, and about fourteene dayes of age, spake certain sencible words, to the wonder of every body.*[10] The "accident" here is an occurrence, but it is more precisely the kind of occurrence that is worth representing to someone else because it is sudden or unexpected. This sense of "accident" as noteworthy event seems quite common in the late sixteenth century. For example, in 1598, J. de Serres produced *An historical collection, of the most memorable accidents, and tragicall massacres of France,* and five years later H. Timberlake used the word in a similar way when he advertised a book describing the "admirable accidents" that "befell" two English pilgrims on their way to Jerusalem.[11]

This broad sense of "accident" as occurrence exists alongside other more precise connotations, but there is no reason to assume that even this generic use of the term did not include our contemporary sense that the accident is "something unforeseen." Several books written in the first decades of the seventeenth century chronicled disastrous "accidents" with hidden or unforeseen causes. Sometimes those disasters were brought about by nature, as this title describes in 1607: *Lamentable newes out of Monmouthshire and Wales. Contayning, the wonderfull and most fearefull accidents of the great overflowing of the waters in the saide county. . . .*[12] The sequel, published the same year, promises the names of ruined towns, the numbers of those lost, and "other reports of accidents that were not before discovered."[13] Such news was also sought abroad. In 1618 a book entitled *Newes from Italy* promises to deliver an account of: *A prodigious and most lamentable accident lately befallen: concerning the swallowing up of the whole citty of Pleurs . . . by a strange and hidious shaking and opening of the earth.*[14] France too had its share of disastrous "accidents." In 1621 *Newes from France* relates "the great losses which happened by the lamentable accident of fire in the citie of Paris," along with the parliamentary decrees designed to "prevent the like mischance in time to come."[15] In this and other early modern texts, the word "chance" is often associated with accidents; here it helps us see that "accident" does not have the generic force of occurrence, but specifically designates an event whose cause could not have been foreseen.

Such unforeseen accidents were just as newsworthy when they occurred in England, often generating intense curiosity about their providential meaning. In 1620, for example, *A warning for all murderers* describes: *A most rare, strange, and wonderful accident, which by Gods just judgement was brought to passe . . . and showne upon three most wicked persons.*[16] The murders are "revenged" for their secret crime "by a childe of five yeeres old, which was in his mothers wombe, and unborne when the deed was done." The sense that such accidents were not "meere chance" occurrences, in William Perkins's well-worn phrase, but events that revealed God's judgment is common in the early seventeenth century.[17] The Blackfriar's "accident" of 1623 mentioned in the previous chapter, for example, provoked a wave of providential speculation and prompted at least one Protestant writer specifically to rule out attempts to credit the "accident" to "chance." In such cases, the word "accident" did double work, preserving a sense of contingency around the unforeseen occurrence without explicitly invoking the pagan concepts of chance and fortune.

The term "accident" also had various technical meanings in astrology, medicine and philosophy. Astrologers, for example, understood an "accident" to be any event that was caused by the stars.[18] In 1624, G. A. Magini's *A strange and wonderfull prognostication* predicted "those accidents which shall, or at least are likely to happen, as may be conjectured by the rules and directions of astrology."[19] Alternatively, "accident" was used in medical discourse to describe symptoms. In 1625, T. Thayre's *An excellent and best approoved treatise of the plague* contains "the nature, signes, and accidents of the same."[20] Finally, in philosophy the term had the technical meaning of a cause or event that could not be foreseen or explained according to some general rule. We see evidence of this particular usage as early as 1490, in the following description of a woman's death: "[H]ir deth naturalle oughte not to haven comen yet of longe tyme, but by accydente and harde fortune."[21] A better-known example of this use of the word comes from an early Shakespeare play, *Love's Labour's Lost*, where the pedantic Holofernes shows his knowledge of the philosophical meaning of "accident" when he describes how Berowne has "framed a letter to a sequent of the stranger Queen's, which, accidentally or by the way of progression, hath miscarried" (4.2.137–38).[22]

While the usage is not directly related to the subject of this book, the term "accident" also referred to one of the four predicables or modes of belonging described in Aristotle's *Categories* and analyzed in the *Metaphysics*.[23] The word "accident" taken in this sense designated an attribute that was logically unrelated to the substance it belonged to—what the Scholastic tradition would describe as that which inheres in a subject, but which could cease to exist without the subject's ceasing to exist as well. This was a crucial concept for early modern theologians analyzing the miracle of the Eucharist, but the theological debates surrounding this definition of "accident" as predicate unfolded along different theological lines than did those surrounding accidental events. In the Eucharist debates, the concept of an "accidental" predicate helped theologians isolate a potentially miraculous substance in the host, whereas in discussions of accidental events, the term focused attention on the generative causes of a temporally unfolding event.[24]

Despite broad use of the term, accidents constituted a recognizable subgroup of contingent events for which any foreseeable natural or human cause was lacking, but which were not miraculous either. It was these events, the apparent purposes they served, and the causes that brought them about that came under renewed scrutiny during the early modern period, in part because Reformation theology raised these issues to a new level of importance. Not only had Calvin's theory of special providence asserted that God was conspicuously active in every unexpected turn of events, but the Protestant insistence that the age of miracles had ceased gave accidents and "contingencies" an increased value as expressions of God's worldly action.[25] As the theologian Thomas Gataker argued, "casualties" can be a direct expression of God's will precisely because their natural causes are so minute; they are divine and natural at the same time.[26] Changing conceptions of causation would also have made accidental events more curious to the philosophically minded: Bacon's theory of forms, for example, transformed accidents from an intellectual dead end into an occasion for discovery—even a model for the experiment itself. Contemporary interest in natural anomalies, such as monsters, prodigies, and the "jokes of nature," moreover, established a realm of "epistemic things" that the category of the accident might help explain.[27]

On an experiential level, life in London around the turn of the seventeenth century would also have encouraged active reflection on accidental events: the flood of individuals mixing randomly in the city would have made unexpected encounters in the streets or in the marketplace an inescapable fact of cosmopolitan life.[28] An emerging merchant economy would have thrived on such a welter of bodies in motion, since it meant that buyers and sellers were capable of circulating in the public spaces of the city at ever greater speeds, presumably to engage in ever more lucrative transactions. The possibility of civic disaster, meanwhile, would never have been far from urban consciousness, a consciousness that habitually framed accidents and mishaps in theatrical terms. As Keith Thomas has noted, London was an extremely dangerous place in which to live in the sixteenth and seventeenth centuries. In a city that lacked an effective fire brigade but was full of wooden structures, a moment's carelessness with lamp or candle could end in "tragedy."[29] Finally, as more and more English merchants "adventured" their fortunes abroad, news of ships being wrecked by tempest or worse—waylaid by a sudden encounter with pirates—would have transformed the sea into a zone of chances, a place in the cultural imagination for accidental occasions or sudden turns of fortune.[30]

Clearly there were other traditions besides the learned one that sustained and enriched this lively early modern encounter with contingency in both its philosophical and material forms. Perhaps the most obvious of these is *Fortuna,* or Fortune, the pagan goddess and poetic abstraction whose resurgence in early modern iconography and poetic imagery has been extensively documented over the course of this century.[31] Gendered female because of her unpredictability, Fortune presided as a deity over the seas and war but could also be invoked as the cause of any outcome that could not be predicted in advance.[32] The literary and philosophical appeal of Fortune stems, in part, from her capacity to become the object of an address: because it is she who sends the storms, she who trips the man in battle, Fortune assumes the narrative position of an agent or actor who can be credited with events that have no immediate organizing cause.[33] This agent is not simply a quasi-mechanical entity that stands in allegorically for some abstract principle that must be systematically unfolded.[34] When viewed as a narrative device, the trope of Fortune also represents the potentially inscrutable nature of causation in a real or imagined world: to the extent that causes are not available for inspection in a particular narrative context—indeed, to the extent that they do not need to be—Fortune can stand in for some pervasive agency outside the narrative frame that guides the fateful paths of ships, individuals or weapons.

The gendered rhetoric of Fortune is one that was particularly appealing to early modern writers. A representative image comes from

Niccolo Machiavelli, who writes in *The Prince* that Fortune is a woman who can be subdued only by bold, decisive action.[35] Machiavelli's rhetoric of subjugating Fortune, one that admittedly contains moments of pragmatic submission, is echoed later on in the work of Francis Bacon, who attempts to tame Fortune and chance in his experimental program by assimilating them into a more masculine form of assertiveness. The rhetorical fulcrum for this transformation of accident into an occasion for action is the notion that accidental events or contingencies are really outcomes that can be performed by a deliberating human (male) agent who shares the drives and desires of the ancient female goddess.[36] Such a tendency to identify an event as a deed and then to infer its doer is often described by Christian writers as an irresistible habit, one which must be carefully managed so that it leads the believer toward God rather than his pagan counterpart. Representing accidents as actions, however, severs their connection with a more subtle form of order—the kind that emerges in the coordination of autonomous world-bound causes rather than the sudden intervention of some deity. Fortune thus represents a potential type for handling accidental events in narrative: to the extent that "she" or "it" can serve as an independent locus of control, the kind of order or purpose expressed in a given narrative world can be triangulated from within. Chance and accident become the effects of an agent who is ultimately like other agents, working with and in the created space of fiction (albeit with supernatural powers), instead of commanding that space from the outside.

When we turn to the romance, a genre characterized by hair's-breadth escapes, wandering siblings, shipwrecks, storms and unexpected encounters, we find the full array of contingent or accidental events that were habitually attributed to Fortune. The first book of Sidney's "Old" *Arcadia* opens with a reference to how Musidorus and Pyrocles were called to meet Euarchus in Byzantium but were forced to detour into Lydia by a tempest. Here, as in the later version of Sidney's prose romance (which opens with another version of shipwreck), the unexpected detour is only the first in a long series of accidents and contingencies variously credited to Fortune or to God.[37] This trope of an accidental encounter at sea, so pervasive in the romance tradition, illustrates a larger structural principle that governs romance action: here accidents and chance encounters are not an interruption of the regular order of things but rather an integral part of a landscape which is obliged to supply them for the purposes of advancing the plot.[38] When Florimell arrives at the seashore just in time to meet the mariner who will carry her away from her lusting pursuer in *The Faerie Queene*, the event unfolds as predictably as the rhyme scheme in one of Spenser's stanzas.[39] Indeed, the almost formal quality of this kind of "necessary" meeting might be described as rhyme on the order of plot, a feature that becomes more obvious when the encounter occurs in verse. Readers experience the happy consonance of means and ends in this scene as a felicitous musical cadence, one that is also a signature or token of some pervasive mode of providential action.

The metaphysical texture of the romance genre, then, makes the accident something organic, the consequence of a landscape whose hills and valleys are guaranteed to bring different characters together at specific times and places. Instead of functioning as sudden interruptions, accidents become a guarantee of smooth narrative transitions. Florimell's unexpected encounter with the mariner confirms a reader's sense that some guiding providence is immanent in the world; the misdelivered letter from the friar in *Romeo and Juliet*, on the other hand, or Dogberry's hapless discovery of Don John's deception in *Much Ado About Nothing*, suggest that contingency is more autonomous and so more genuinely disruptive. Unlike in the romance, the pathos or humor of accident in these plays would fade if characters or objects (like the letter) lost their autonomy and instead became puppets in some larger moral or allegorical scheme. This is not to dismiss the romance representation of chance and accident as fake or unreal, but rather to show that different genres embody alternative presuppositions about the relationship between agents and the world in which they act—about known causes and their purchase on the created world of fiction. In the case of the romance, those causes are not sufficiently independent to generate the curiosity and surprise, much less the sense of metaphysical paradox, that surrounds accidents in other genres.

Fortune makes accident a personified form of action; romance buries the accident in a world in which it is no exception: in both cases, the accident as contingent, spontaneous event slowly disappears or becomes something else. When we turn to the rhetorical-legal tradition, we find that the real possibility of accidents—one recognized by the law—is actualized only when the art of narration is properly employed. As early as Cicero, we find in the *De inventione* that a criminal act may be admitted but then excused if one pleads that it was done by chance [*casus*]. In such cases, Cicero points out that the orator or advocate must narrate the event in such a way that its accidental character will become clear. Similar statements appear in the *Rhetorica ad Herennium*, and we know that both of these texts helped shape judicial pleading through the early modern period.[40] One outgrowth of that tradition—the Ramist reforms in dialectic and logic—continued to identify accidental causes and accidental events as indispensable topics for the invention of arguments. In his *Logic*, for example, Ramus preserves the genus of accidental efficient cause (explicated with literary examples) in a way that harks back to Cicero's treatment of the topic. Under the heading of Efficient Cause in his first book, he writes: "By accident the cause workethe, which by some externall power workethe, as in those thinges whiche are done by necessitie, or by fortune."[41] An effect can be the result of "necessity"—and so be produced by "accident"—when an intending agent is prevented from determining the outcome of his actions. "Fortune," moreover, "is a cause by accident, when besides the intente of the worker, some other thing chauncethe." Ignorance and lack of foresight are both signs that the accidental cause of Fortune is at work in the realm of human actions. Ramus's mixture of chance and fortune under the heading of accidental efficient cause is clearly an Aristotelian inheritance, as are several of the technical terms here (chance, accident, fortune, necessity). While I will be working to explicate these terms more carefully below, the presence of such distinctions in what was once the rhetorical office of invention alerts us to the fact that the accidental cause was still recognized as a good "place" to look for arguments in the sixteenth century.

English law also made specific provisions for pardoning unintentional or accidental criminal acts, particularly homicide.[42] Although the distinction between manslaughter and murder would alter these categories in the sixteenth century, the kinds of homicide that might be pardoned as accidental are worth noting. Accidents involving carts drawn by horses, those involving plows, and those involving guns and archers might all be pardoned because they were not deliberate acts. Some of the most difficult cases to decide involved fights, since one had to differentiate self-defense, which was an intentional killing of sorts, from accidental killing—the latter being granted when an assailant was seen to have "fallen" on the stationary weapon of the accused.[43]

Because the English law required a *mens rea,* or malicious intent, to assign guilt, the plea that something had been done by accident was effective because it eliminated the defendant's intention from the possible causes of an event.[44] Unlike the tradition of romance or Fortune, the legal tradition of dealing with accidents was very much interested in seeking the cause for such events in human intentions. When the defendant's intention could be ruled out as a cause, Green shows that other agents — the deceased, or in some cases an animal — were blamed for the outcome.[45] This focus on human agents and intentions persisted even when it was clear that the accused had had no plan to commit a given act. Luke Wilson analyzes the case of a man trying to poison his wife but instead poisoning his daughter, showing how a fictional intention could be "attached" to the accidental act and so bring it back under the purview of the law.[46] We see some of the complexities of this style of reasoning in *Hamlet* when the gravedigger parodies the legal language surrounding Ophelia's death.

In the rhetorical-legal tradition, accidents become a real class of events with a distinctly narrative pedigree: to the extent that narrative description can detach such occurrences from a particular intention or person (usually by focusing on intervening circumstances), certain actions become events and so acquire special status under the law. Philosophy also isolates the accident as a class of events: like unforeseen outcomes that cannot be called crimes, accidents are outcomes that cannot be subsumed under a regular rule. Cicero's rhetorical advice carries over here, since in order to detach accidents from other rule-bound phenomena, philosophers must often give a narrative account of the particular circumstances in which they occur. Aristotle, for example, isolates accidents as a distinct class of events by focusing on their particular causes — causes that must ultimately be called out for inspection in a quasi-narrative description. Aristotle's analysis, which furnishes the learned tradition with a set of examples that it can mull over and elaborate, makes accidents the result of an unexpected meeting of independent causal chains.[47] One could not make any general link between the contributing causes themselves and the particular accidental effects they might produce. In the *Metaphysics*, for example, he describes a ship's having been met by pirates as an example of something that has come about by accident: "Going to Aegina was an accident, if the man went not in order to get there, but because he was carried out of his way by a storm or captured by pirates."[48]

The effect of this analysis is to remove Fortune as a spontaneous agent of such "actions" and instead render them as events that could not be foreseen by any deliberating agent. As events, accidents would require a different rhetoric and conceptual scheme from the one used to render such occurrences as the actions of an abstract agency like Fortune. Confluence, coincidence, meeting, and joining were the preferred terms for characterizing these occurrences, and the use of them created a causal vacuum where the goddess *Fortuna* once was. For Aristotle, this vacuum was not worth fearing, since the point in dealing with accidents was to recognize that they were events instead of actions. As we will see in the next chapter, Aristotle's analysis made it possible to eliminate the middle-woman when discussing such events, a possibility subsequent Christian thinkers exploited when they delivered her duties to an omnipotent male God.

The Aristotelian Analysis of Accidents

Aristotle's impulse is always to think about accidents as a problem, singling them out as an exception to the rules that govern change in the world. Underlying this impulse to isolate accidents is a desire to limit their disruptive power. If accidents have causes and express purposes in the same way that other events or actions do, Aristotle recognizes, then concepts like cause and purpose become difficult to maintain in a larger metaphysical scheme. More broadly, if accidental events really are not exceptions to the rule of regular causation (a possibility I will explore below), it becomes impossible to anchor human knowledge in a set of metaphysical causes, so named because they act in a regular way. Accidents are thus subjected to a kind of epistemological hygiene in various Aristotelian texts. Unless they are emptied of metaphysical content, readers are told, they offer endless opportunities for confusion. It is not surprising, then, to find Aristotle suggesting that "accident" is a mere name, what Hamlet would call a "windy suspiration of forcéd breath." "[We] must first say regarding the accidental, that there can be no scientific treatment of it," he states categorically in the *Metaphysics*.[49] But the topic gets extended treatment nevertheless.

If we want eventually to grasp the narrative and cultural significance of accidents under Aristotle's description, we must do so indirectly, through an analysis of his arguments for their exclusion from metaphysics. Those arguments follow from a series of comparisons which isolate the accident as a category of event, usually with reference to other events that are determined by regularly acting metaphysical causes. In the *Physics*, for example, he argues that because accidental events have accidental causes, they can be opposed to other events that have intrinsic ones: "For just as a thing is something either in virtue of itself or accidentally, so may it be a cause. For instance, the house-building faculty is in virtue of itself a cause of the house, whereas the pale or the musical is an accidental cause."[50] Just as substances can be connected to their attributes in various ways, Aristotle is saying, causal agents can be connected in various ways to their effects. Some attributes of the agent, for example, his or her paleness, may be unrelated to the agent's ability to produce a given effect, whereas others (the ability to build) are crucial.[51] Accidental events are thus not produced by an intrinsic cause which acts in a regular and self-sufficient way. Rather, as Susan Sauvé Meyer explains, accidental events "simply result" and are indifferent to the purposes that the great variety of agents have determined (naturally or voluntarily) to bring about in the world.[52]

When Aristotle considers what it is that becomes an accidental cause in the *Physics*, he decides that it must be one of those efficient causes which produce change in the world—causes that alter matter and in doing so realize or destroy what is potential in it. Aristotle mentions several kinds of efficient causes at work in the sublunar realm: the will, nature, and two accidental causes that in common speech are referred to as chance (*automaton,* usually translated into Latin as *casus*) and fortune (*tuche,* which for the most part is rendered by *fortuna* in Latin).[53] There is a hierarchy among these causes. The will and nature are intrinsic or *per se* causes: as long as they are not impeded, they are sufficient to bring about their effects without aid of another cause. Such effects are brought about both in human affairs and in nature, realms in which things are done "for the sake of something." When a house-builder builds a house, he is the *per se* efficient cause of what he builds. Similarly, an oak tree has a *per se* cause in nature that regularly brings fully formed oak trees from acorns. What we see in both these cases are teleological processes in which *per se* causes act in predictable ways to bring about recognizable purposes.

For Aristotle there is a crucial link between the regularity of certain events in nature and their purposiveness: to the extent that certain things happen most or all of the time—acorns giving rise to oak trees rather than palms—we know that such happenings have come about for a reason. Indeed, to speak of a nature or essence at all is, for Aristotle, to assume that such a nature has the power to do things the same way in most cases, and that this "doing" is in the service of some goal.

Because it is in some ways regular, the world proves susceptible to metaphysical analysis in terms of the natural "kinds" at work in nature. Individuals and living organisms have the power to do things in a certain way, and that particular way of working is knowable to the extent that it is general. This kind of nut gives rise to this tree, Aristotle would say, and in invoking kinds, he isolates the aspects of natural processes that can be generalized to support organized forms of inference and deduction. The workings of the will, moreover, are related to the causally determined regularity which is at the foundation of Aristotle's scheme. To the extent that the will can actually be said to cause an outcome, Aristotle would argue, it must be aiming at that particular outcome. If you want an oak tree, you plant an acorn: the punctuality of certain events in the world is thus what lets the will "take aim" at outcomes in a purposive way.

Because wills and natural causes are independent of one another, however, they can join unexpectedly, producing outcomes that are not determined by an individual *per se* cause.[54] Such joinings are rare, but they occur in the realms of nature and deliberate action—the same realms where the *per se* causes work to bring about purposive results. In such cases the event may seem to serve a purpose, even when none of the agents that brought it about had that specific purpose in mind. The effects of these joinings are said to occur "by accident" (*kata sumbebekos*, or the Latin, *per accidens*). Meeting, joining, or falling into place are all terms used to describe the process whereby two or more independent causal chains meet and become the accidental causes of events that might have been aimed at deliberately.[55] When such events happen, the underpinnings of Aristotle's metaphysical scheme have to be reasserted, which he does by demonstrating the arbitrary quality of the causes and purposes which are assigned to these events.

Several examples are offered to illustrate accidental events that are commonly called chance or fortune, many of which involve literal meetings or falling. Book Two of the *Physics* supplies the following, which may have been taken from comedies popular in Aristotle's time: "Example: A man is engaged in collecting subscriptions for a feast. He would have gone to such and such a place for the purpose of getting the money, if he had known. He actually went there for another purpose, and it was only accidentally that he got his money by going there."[56] Now some, who believe that accidents really are determined by a *per se* cause, use a similar example to argue their point. They say that "coming by chance into the market and finding there a man whom one wanted but did not expect to meet is due to one's wish to go and buy in the market."[57] Aristotle will agree that it was necessary for the man to have such a wish for the meeting to occur, but that wish was not the *per se* cause of the meeting; rather, it was the accidental one. I will try to explain this difference more fully after looking at a few more examples. It is important to recognize here, however, that for Aristotle it is the meeting or joining of the two men that needs to be explained. One cannot say that the man's wish to go to the market is the cause of that meeting without qualification. This kind of accident is an example of what Aristotle describes as *tuche*—the accidental cause that works in and through agents capable of deliberation (sane, adult humans). Here is another of the same kind, taken from the *Metaphysics*: "We call an accident that which attaches to something and can be truly asserted, but neither of necessity nor usually, e.g. if one in digging a hole for a plant found treasure. This—the finding of treasure—happens by accident to the man who digs the hole."[58]

Digging holes or plowing rarely leads to treasure, and so finding that treasure cannot have been the result of a deliberate act. We can extend the idea with an early modern example. When the once wealthy hero Timon in Shakespeare's *Timon of Athens* begins to dig for roots near his cave, he is not looking for the treasure he discovers there, and perhaps would *not* have dug for it had he known what he would find. (Timon has forsworn wealth and so is in the ironic position of not wanting the "good" that accidentally comes his way.) Finding the treasure is thus an accident with respect to the cause of digging: Timon's desire to find roots. In offering the example of buried treasure, Aristotle maintains that there is a link between what one expects and what one tries deliberately to get. You plow because it makes farming easier, go to the market because—usually—you can find grapes or oil there. Natural processes, the habits, reasons and customs of others, inasmuch as they are regular, all become the objects of deliberation in this way.

There are many other purposes besides finding gold which accidental events can satisfy. Elsewhere in the *Physics*, Aristotle writes: "We say, for instance, that a stranger has come by chance, paid the ransom, and gone away, when he does so as if he had come for that purpose, though it was not for that that he came. This is accidental, for chance is an accidental cause, as I remarked before."[59] The example is vague enough to seem like the kind of thing that does happen once in a while, but of course Aristotle wants to avoid giving the impression that such "ransomings" are an abstract class of events with a common cause. As with other examples of accidental events, this one serves to point out that the accident is a dead end for causal reasoning, since the causes of accidents are indefinite. What does indefinite mean here? Practically speaking, one could come up with any number of versions of the above story in which the accidental payment of the ransom would have happened: it does not matter what the particular cause of ransoming was as long as there was a ransom to be paid. The fact that we can substitute any reason for going to the place where the ransom might be paid shows that the outcome is indifferent to the kind of purposes that accidentally produce it—indifferent, that is, in the logical or metaphysical sense. The accident is an event which does not follow of metaphysical necessity from the particular desires and actions of those who have brought it about.

What is nevertheless interesting about accidents—and Aristotle seems aware of this fact—is that they are still necessary in some less-than-metaphysical way. Given the ship headed into the unforeseen storm, the two people headed to the same stall in the market, we can see that the outcome could not have been otherwise. Aristotle's point is that there is no metaphysical reason why things could not have been otherwise in such cases, only circumstantial or "accidental" ones. Whatever "gives" the particulars which make the accident inevitable, that "giver" is not constrained to do so by laws that a philosopher could discover. Susan Suavé Meyer, in her analysis of Aristotle's treatment of accidents, makes the distinction between the determination of an outcome by its causes and the overdetermination of that outcome.[60] This distinction may help clarify the difference between the two types of necessity Aristotle is describing. A *per se* cause is recognizable because it overdetermines its effects. That is to say, the proper action of a *per se* cause will not be impeded by any number of differences in "circumstances." There are entire classes of circumstances that can be bracketed in advance, allowed to vary in an indefinite array of possible worlds, without affecting the power of the *per se* cause to determine its effects.[61] Rain can be expected from thunder clouds regardless of the phase of the moon. But a *per se* cause working accidentally does not overdetermine its effects in this way; rather, it just determines them. Given the circumstances, this particular man's trip to the market for grapes has put him on a collision course with this other man who is going there for oil. There is no general link, however, between going to the market for oil and meeting one's debtors. The crucial accident of their meeting cannot be seen to follow of necessity—say, in some future instance—from the particular kind of desires that led these people to the market in the first place.

There are several other examples of *tuche* or deliberating agents producing accidental results that I will mention before moving on to *automaton*. Two are of "good" outcomes produced accidentally—for example, when a confectioner manages to produce something that is both sweet and healthful.[62] The other example of this kind is that of a man who becomes healthy after a haircut, not because his hair is shorter but because the sun he was exposed to while getting the haircut was good for his health.[63] Health is an obvious accidental good for Aristotle, just as gold was in the plowing example mentioned above. Of course, bad things can happen accidentally as well. One example that seems already to be part of philosophical lore is the case in which a man eats pungent food, becomes thirsty, and is killed by bandits when he goes outside to get a drink.[64] Aristotle cites the example in order to refute the idea that the fortuitous event can be traced back indefinitely through a chain of preceding causes. In other words, the man does not die because of the food he ate. The cause of his death seems, rather, to be his unexpected meeting with those who would kill him, and it is at this joining where one must stop when tracing back the causes of the man's death.[65]

We have now seen enough examples to distinguish between what Aristotle called *tuche* (luck or fortune) and *automaton* (chance). *Tuche* refers to that class of accidental events that result from agents capable of deliberation, while *automaton* is a term for what befalls nondeliberating agents.[66] An example of *tuche* would be the man who sets out on a sea journey, deliberately determining to go to one place, but whose course changes accidentally because he meets pirates or a tempest along the way. By contrast, Aristotle points to the situation in which a tripod falls spontaneously and lands in such a position that it might serve as a seat.[67] Because tripods are not deliberating beings, this outcome is a species of chance or *automaton*. Another example: "We say, for example, that the horse came spontaneously, because, though his coming saved him, he did not come for the sake of safety."[68] Because a horse is not capable of rational deliberation (according to Aristotle), the horse's safety is said to be brought about by chance. Finally, Aristotle describes a rock that falls and kills a man—something the stone in no way "wanted" to do, but which someone might have deliberately done by throwing that stone at the man.[69] In differentiating these two realms, Aristotle is in part trying to account for common uses of the words *tuche* and *automaton*, showing that they point to a real distinction among the kinds of agents (deliberating, nondeliberating) that can become accidental causes. But his discussion of *automaton* also communicates the sense in which, at least in the case of the tripod or the stone, the brute necessity of matter falling downward is capable of bringing a purposive outcome about. In a way, even deliberating agents are transformed into this kind of matter-in-motion when an accident happens, not because they are suddenly emptied of intelligence on such occasions, but because it is their mere presence in a particular place—a body that arrives in this locale rather than some other at the right moment—which enables the accidental outcome to occur automatically.

What is paramount for Aristotle in all of these examples is that we do not put the causes of accidental outcomes in the wrong place. If, for instance, we observe the falling tripod and assert that it has an intrinsic power to fall in the position of a seat, Aristotle would say that we have extended the characteristics of its "kind" improperly. Following this logic, we might say that the art of house-building is responsible for domestic arguments, because house-builders create the places where such arguments occur. But this assertion—that all the effects of a particular cause are intrinsically related to that cause—would then allow us to credit the house-builder with any of a potentially unlimited number of the outcomes that his craft enables. If a peace treaty is signed in that particular house, it was thanks to the house-builder. If a murder occurs in that house as a result of a domestic dispute, the house-builder was responsible. The sheer number of outcomes that can be attached to the act of building the house is what makes a concept like the "accidental" indispensable: it prevents an analysis from slipping into the realm of the "indeterminate," where the number of possible effects for a cause is potentially infinite.

In the above examples, Aristotle's use of the accidental cause is consistently applied to preserve the domain of *per se* causation. One of the most controversial areas of Aristotle's invocation of accidental causes, however, is in his analysis of the generation of living beings, an area where nature is understood to reproduce kind from kind in a regular, purposive fashion. Sometimes a thing is produced "in vain" or "contrary to nature," he writes in the *Physics*, and in such monstrous cases we see nature deviating from the usual purposes that it strives unconsciously to meet.[70] Aristotle includes these instances because they are said to be brought about by chance (*automaton*), but never by fortune (*tuche*), and in doing so he may simply be acknowledging a common use of the term *automaton*.[71] There is not a neat fit, however, between things that are "contrary to nature" and the other chance events which Aristotle has been analyzing. To begin with, Aristotle's previous examples of chance events do not emphasize the frustration of a purpose, but the unanticipated completion of one. Further complicating matters is the fact that monsters or natural deviants seem to have a *per se* cause rather than an accidental one because they have an intrinsic—or at least, internal—principle of determination.[72] Aristotle seems to anticipate the latter criticism at least when he says that things "contrary to nature" are not really part of the category of *automaton* proper, "for the cause of the latter is external, that of the former internal." The discussion is a vexed one, however, and is not resolved in the various readings of this passage offered by Aristotle's commentators.[73]

The ambiguity of Aristotle's discussion of chance events in nature with an internal cause is an enabling one, since his treatment of things "contrary to nature" allows subsequent thinkers to include monsters and natural deviants in their discussion of the general class of events that occur by accident.[74] The linkage will be crucial for Francis Bacon in Chapter four, when he characterizes monsters as a spontaneous expression of artifice in nature, thereby strengthening the link between "accidental" productions and a hidden form of craft that those productions might reveal. The example of things "contrary" to nature demonstrates, moreover, the difficulty of preserving the process of *per se* causation entirely within natural processes of development. Where cause and effect work within a living being, conjoined in a womb instead of in the marketplace or at sea, the distinction between intrinsic and extrinsic becomes difficult for Aristotle to maintain. And yet, he seems committed to the usefulness of the term "accident" in such cases, since it clearly identifies what is "contrary to nature" as part of that exceptional category of events with no *per se* cause; so described, they need not be accounted for in causal terms, and the link between cause and regularity in the rest of nature is preserved.

The examples and analysis provided above illustrate what Aristotle has to lose if he fails to isolate accidents as a special (and ultimately insignificant) case of events in the world: without this category, the possible causes of a given event become innumerable, the intrinsic purposiveness of natural processes and voluntary acts ceases to be assured, and the broader link between regularity and abstract, knowable "kinds" begins to dissolve. Given the stakes, his unwillingness to assign accidents a metaphysical cause is understandable. But what is the value of the category that results from Aristotle's extended exercise in intellectual housekeeping? How does his precise sense of what an accident is help us think about other issues which may not have been his immediate concern? As the irrational exception that proves the rule, the accident points us away from metaphysics toward a scene in which cultural value is recognized and reproduced.

Consider first the purposes which accidents are seen to serve in Aristotle's discussion. A man who is plowing a field stumbles upon buried treasure and is enriched as a result. Had he known that the treasure was there, he would have dug for it deliberately, but since he did not, we consider this goal hypothetically: given the way things turned out, it was "as if" he were doing the plowing to find the treasure. But what if the man turned up a set of fish bones, some leaves, or an old piece of rusted iron instead?[75] What is turned up "by accident" is not just some goodie, but a network of assumptions about what is good, bad, worthwhile, or purposeful. "I wanted the treasure in general," the farmer might say, "but not at that moment." For the farmer to identify a purpose that he had but did not have, he has to reach into a communal reservoir of intentions and purposes that were somehow already there, waiting to be satisfied—a solution of suspended ends that the accident precipitates into a single moment of satisfaction. Aristotle's example of an accident only becomes an example, then, when it is offered in a context where the acquisition of lost treasure is generally understood to be valuable.

This is hardly a trivial point. While the various goods cited in Aristotle's examples seem obvious (health, safety, riches, repayment), they are nonetheless contingent on culturally specific notions of value. Consider now the more complicated case of a man's being accidentally killed by the falling of a stone. Death or killing are sometimes pursued deliberately, which is what makes this particular outcome an example of an accident. But the "purposive" nature of the outcome is not simply the person's being killed. If the deceased was an inveterate atheist, flouting the Gods at every turn, the accident will seem to have come about "as if" it were a divine form of punishment. To whom will it seem so? To those who share the assumption that the Gods jealously protect their authority. The more elaborate a particular culture's views are on the nature of death, revenge, the Gods or riches, the more likely it is that accidental events involving these factors will be identified as such. When the Elizabethan audience of *Hamlet* hears Horatio's final reference to "casual slaughters," for example, it is being forced to actively engage its own communal assumptions about the contradictory purposes or "ends" that shape life and death: the dramatic power of Horatio's words would fade if those assumptions were monolithic or sequestered in some perfectly isolated spectatorial consciousness.

Aristotle has isolated a spurious kind of goal or *telos*—what we might call the hypothetical purpose of accident—which can serve as a model for the kind of value that circulates in a given culture, value which individual members can attach to events without, so to speak, being prompted. How does such value get linked to the spontaneous events that express them? The process is one of narrative description. When we look at Aristotle's analysis of accidents in books like the *Physics* and the *Metaphysics*, we find again and again that the only way to explain an accidental event is to tell a story about it. Some of these stories are only sketched—for example, a man plowing a field unexpectedly finds treasure—but in every one of them there is an implied beginning, middle and end. Take the example cited early on in the *Physics* of the man who unexpectedly comes into money:

> A man is engaged in collecting subscriptions for a feast. He would have gone to such and such a place for the purpose of getting the money, if he had known. He actually went there for another purpose, and it was only accidentally that he got his money by going there.

What makes this example a story is the fact that, in addition to describing the itinerary of a particular person, it describes the arc of an intention and its modification. Taking a break from his attempts to raise money for a feast, a man goes to the market to buy grapes, but then encounters an old friend who is able to give him a contribution. The initial intention of buying grapes (beginning) has been "crossed" by an unexpected meeting (middle) that results in the satisfaction of a pre-existing desire (end). Aristotle's examples of encounters with pirates at sea or robbers at the well could be expanded in similar terms; in each case, we would see that a sequence of actions becomes a story at precisely the moment when an intention to do one thing undergoes alteration.

Here we can make another nonmetaphysical observation: stories about accidents invite readers to think about intentions as if they were "trajectories" of persons or objects, and then watch as something "happens" to that trajectory, not literally, but as an extension of the objects involved. The intention to keep treasure hidden, for example, "sits" buried in the chest underground. The intention to plant crops, alternatively, is "carried" along the path of the plow. At some point, the path of the plow intersects with the location of the chest. What happened? It is not simply the case that bodies in motion have collided: intentions have met and crossed as well. We can extend this observation by saying that narrative itself is a kind of "shuttle" for intentions that are subject to change—like the boat which carries the hapless passenger into the path of pirates. To the extent that readers or spectators do not know what is in store for them, they are like the person on the ship headed to Aegina or the farmer making furrows with a plow. (Indeed, it is on this basis that they may identify with such a character.) Only when that trajectory is interrupted—when "something happens" to the expectations that are bound up in a particular path of action—is the story really under way.[76]

Returning to the metaphysical analysis of accidents in Aristotle's philosophy, we can say that the "empty status" of these events with respect to *per se* causes is exactly what qualifies them for explanation through narrative exposition. Aristotle's rendering of accidents as simply determined or metaphysically indifferent makes them moments when particularity and circumstances have real determining power. Yes, there may be details that could have remained the same without changing the outcome itself—say if the man who goes to the market has brown eyes instead of blue.[77] But if that same man had stopped along the way to the market to fix his sandal and, so, missed the wealthy friend he otherwise would have met, we get a sense of the fragility of the meeting itself. It matters that the event turned out one way instead of another, and accounting for this kind of particularity-without-overdetermination—the fact that circumstances were "just so" in a particular case—is a matter of saying how things were, not of citing general rules.

Philosophy must pass over this kind of simple determination of events in silence, since mere circumstantial necessity provides no foothold for inference or generalization. But narrative is built on this kind of circumstantial explanation: a story can set out what happened as a result of this man's trip to the market without citing a general rule; the storyteller simply describes the man's arrival at one end of the market and then tells us that, quite unexpectedly, his friend has appeared at the other end. Narrative thus trades on what Aristotle identifies as our less-than-metaphysical knowledge of circumstances, giving us (and characters) a partial view of how things stand and then playing on those limitations. If stories are built on circumstantial knowledge in this way, then stories become the privileged means by which one represents an accident as a contingent event. Aristotle's category of the accident helps us understand why narrative can fulfill this role in the explanation of accidents when metaphysics cannot: accidents happen as the result of circumstances, not rules, and only narrative can lay out these circumstances as a matter of fact rather than a function of overdetermining causes. This discussion also suggests that, given the kind of knowledge one has of circumstances (a limited knowledge of contingent facts), there is no exalted form of understanding being unearthed by readers who follow a story to find out "what happens." The knowledge one has of an accident, according to Aristotle, is simply a knowledge of what happened. If there is a secret lying buried in the treasure chest, it is only the secret of where the chest is buried.

The idea that accidents put individuals in touch with only the slenderest knowledge of circumstances will be reversed in the early modern period when Calvin and his interpreters assert that accidents reveal the astonishing sweep of God's providence. Within natural philosophy, Bacon will make a parallel claim when he points out that accidents have the power to "discover" a hidden order in nature that would otherwise go unnoticed. Aristotle's discussion prepares us to appreciate the magnitude of this early modern shift, but it also articulates the conditions under which such a transformation is possible. There is something about poetic fiction in general and tragic drama in particular—the realm of things which might be—that allows accidents to assume some legitimate purposive quality that they are denied in metaphysics. Placing accidents in a fictional frame, precisely what Calvin and his English interpreters do when they popularize the theatrical metaphor in the late sixteenth century, is thus for Aristotle a means of putting that hypothetical purpose of the accident to legitimate use.

Aristotle explicitly states that accidents have legitimate meaning and power on stage in his discussion of complex plots in the *Poetics,* where he criticizes episodic plots in which "there is neither probability nor necessity in the sequence of its episodes" (1451b35). Aristotle opposes this kind of plot to that which is appropriate for Tragedy, saying:

> Tragedy, however, is an imitation not only of a complete action, but also of incidents arousing pity and fear. Such incidents have the very greatest effect on the mind when they occur unexpectedly and at the same time in consequence of one another; there is more of the marvelous in them than if they happened of themselves or by mere chance. Even matters of chance seem most marvelous if there is an appearance of design as it were in them; as for instance the statue of Mitys at Argos killed the author of Mitys' death by falling down on him when he was looking at it; for incidents like that we think to be not without a meaning. A plot, therefore, of this sort is necessarily finer than others.[78]

The meaning expressed in the murderer's death here stems more from the spatial pattern of events rather than a linear sequence of cause and effect. It is not the cause of the statue's motion that imparts a larger sense of purpose to the outcome, but the fact that the murderer happens to be standing just underneath it. This purpose-in-position is obviously different from the kinds of purposes that Aristotle associates with *per se* causation above. The poetic effect described here could not be accomplished if, say, a deliberating agent pushed the statue from above (a form of violent motion), nor if it was destined by nature to fall only on that particular man (a perversion of Aristotle's natural motion).

When Aristotle admits that the accident acquires a qualified meaning on stage, the hypothetical purpose of such events becomes a virtue instead of a liability. Indeed, what he describes as poetic "meaning"—still an indispensable category for literary and cultural criticism—becomes far richer for both literary studies and intellectual history when it is equated with the spurious purpose of accidental events. Such a parallel allows us to realize that drama and other genres of fiction encapsulate an inarticulate "metaphysics" or set of organizing assumptions about how the totality of events in a given world are related to some hypothetical source of order.[79] The comparison of this fictional kind of order with another that governs the world at large, one that I have to a certain degree forced on Aristotle, would have been almost intuitive in the early modern period. In his *Apology for Poetry,* for example, Philip Sidney describes the order of fiction as a "pattern" manifest in the sequence of events, one that can be imposed by the poet but cannot be manipulated by the historian. Elsewhere in the *Apology* he develops this comparison by saying that while history must be overruled by fortune, poetry can "frame" events and examples according to an ideal type.[80] One writer invents, the other records. Such comparisons support crucial ontological distinctions, distinctions that emerge most sharply when a writer like Sidney tries to specify the kind of order or purpose which ought to be ascribed to accidental events in different narrative frames.

But Aristotle's discussion is really about drama, not "poetry" as a whole, and so this chapter should really end with the theater. Aristotle's analysis suggests that the theater generalizes conditions that surround accidents in the world, which is why accidents cease to have an exceptional status under the arches. Like all events on stage, accidents are laden with another, externally imposed purpose which—if it is not assumed outright—can at least never be demonstrated not to exist. The rock in Aristotle's example thus falls both because it is a rock and because it is responding to the gravitational desires of its theatrical creator (or alternatively, the expectations of the audience that interprets its fall). To view something theatrically is, we might say, to have already agreed that such other purposes and desires exist in the world and that one is in a position to recognize them. Clearly this is what Aristotle was counting on when he delivered the orphaned purposes of accidents to the imaginary world of drama. Those purposes would thrive beyond the confines of the stage in the providentialism of the late sixteenth and seventeenth centuries, but only after Aristotle's assertion that accidents lack any real cause had been squared with the Christian conviction that all events, even accidents, were designed by God.

CHAPTER 2

Exemplary Accidents from Cicero to Jean Calvin

> Human life is beset by innumerable evils, and threatened with a thousand deaths. . . . Embark on a ship; there is but a single step between you and death. Mount a horse; the slipping of one foot endangers your life. Walk through the streets of a city; you are liable to as many dangers as there are tiles on the roofs. If there be a sharp weapon in your hand, or that of your friend, the mischief is manifest. All the ferocious animals you see are armed for your destruction. If you endeavor to shut yourself in a garden surrounded with a good fence, and exhibiting nothing but what is delightful, even there sometimes lurks a serpent.[1]
>
> —Jean Calvin, *Institutes of the Christian Religion*

"There is but a single step between you and death." With this grim warning, Jean Calvin telescopes all of life's uncertainty into a single moment of deliberate action, a fatal step that decides all that is to come. In focusing on the critical moment of transition—stepping onboard the ship that will soon be lost—Calvin joins a long tradition of writers who are attracted to the moment when the unforeseen accident becomes inevitable. While his views on these events differ dramatically from those of his Scholastic predecessors, Calvin's desire to catalogue accidents and to locate their causes in a particular agent, object or occasion is familiar. The individual who takes the portentous step in this example could easily be the man in Aristotle's *Metaphysics*, embarking on a ship bound for Aegina without any idea that pirates will divert him along the way. Like both Aristotle and Calvin, philosophically minded ancient and medieval writers would carefully examine the punctual linkages of intention and action that preceded accidental events. A man enters the marketplace, only to spy his friend. Another, thirsty, goes to the well to drink. Two people meet unexpectedly, and suddenly they have fallen in love. As spectators crowd around it, a statue begins to fall. . . .

The career of such examples and the theories that were adduced to explain them are the subject of this chapter, which briefly surveys the trajectories of falling objects, unexpected meetings at sea, monstrous births and other accidental encounters in texts representing several centuries' worth of speculation on the causes and purposes of accidental events. While there is a case to be made for passage of such examples directly into the texts of early modern writers such as Shakespeare, Calvin and Bacon, my interest here is more genealogical than genetic. By examining the circulation of "exemplary accidents" across divergent analytic frames, I want to take stock of their persistence as a figure of thought in texts by Cicero, Boethius, Augustine, Albert, Aquinas, Oresme and Calvin. The repeated invocation of accidents in these texts suggests that such events posed powerful philosophical questions about causation in an economical form, problems that could be carefully analyzed with the help of examples tailored for the purpose. This capacity of accidents to command the explanatory resources of the tradition derived, ironically enough, from the very qualities that led Aristotle to dismiss them. Because they represented a lapse of intelligible order in the world, accidents became a challenge or test case for anyone wanting to account for that order in a systematic way.

By the time Calvin began writing his *Institutes* in the 1530s, learned discussion of these events had moved well beyond the intellectual confines that Aristotle had set for it. While Aristotle's sense of the accident's definitive metaphysical emptiness remained strong throughout antiquity and into the Middle Ages, Christian writers attempted nevertheless to harmonize it with a new and equally categorical conviction: that God maintains complete control over every act and element in creation. The first intellectually compelling compromise between these two positions was formulated by Boethius, who merged Aristotle's analysis of accident with a Christian theology of God's providence. In doing so, Boethius helped subsequent theologians to embrace the contradictory notion that God foresaw and controlled accidents without taking an active role in bringing them about. The very idea of an accident or accidental cause, however, would be ruthlessly criticized from other quarters during late antiquity. Augustine is perhaps the most influential early member of an opposing, hostile faction—one that would eventually be joined by Calvin in the sixteenth century—arguing that it was a corruption of faith to introduce accidental causes like chance or fortune into an analysis of events which were the immediate works of God.

Calvin had a deep knowledge of this tradition and, perhaps more important, knew that it offered a ready set of examples that could be appropriated for his own purposes of spiritual reform.[2] Throughout his discussion of God's "special providence" in the *Institutes*, the accidents catalogued above are situated in a new theological framework in which God's executive power over creation takes priority over all other aspects of his divine control. God not only knows what will happen, he makes it so in an active, interested way. In using these examples but attributing to them a different significance, Calvin articulates an important shift in sixteenth-century views on the relationship between God and creation.[3] For Calvin and his English interpreters, God would become a doer rather than a surveyor, and accidents would turn out to be a privileged means by which his pervasive presence could be glimpsed. Instead of thinking of creation as an ongoing demonstration of rational divine principles, adherents to the theory of special or particular providence saw it instead as a theater or mirror: by carefully attending to a world in which accidents punished some and rewarded others, individuals might gain experiential knowledge of God's divine presence in the world. This providential view of history and experience would be raised, in England, to the level of a "mode of civic consciousness" in the sixteenth century: not only was it a doctrinal watchword of the Protestant left, but a more general principle for understanding English history.[4] While Calvin urged restraint in interpreting the specific intentions of God's providential will in history, English Protestants would nevertheless spend time looking to their daily lives for signs of God's judgment.[5]

As I have already suggested, such tectonic shifts in the relationship between God, nature and the deliberating human subject are best grasped in the dissemination of the examples discussed in the last chapter. This process takes place directly through textual commentary or indirectly, as new examples of accidents arrive either to eclipse or extend older ones. The falling tripod, the horse that is saved by fleeing, the man who finds his debtor when he goes to the market to buy something: each of these accidents appears unaltered in the texts of Islamic and patristic commentators.[6] But while many such accidents are simply carried over in the process of commentary, some undergo significant changes as they pass from one writer to the next. These divergences in example and argument will serve as the focus of my analysis below, which links several "types" of accident arbitrarily derived from Aristotle—the meeting of ships, unexpected encounters among persons, monstrous births and errant or falling objects—to a revolving set of arguments in classical, medieval and the early modern thought. At times my survey will involve jumping from one historical period to the next, something that is inevitable when dealing with a body of thought elaborated over the course of a millennium. While this approach may result in a somewhat diminished sense of development and progression, the strategy of analyzing "exemplary accidents" has the advantage of showing precisely how mobile these examples were in the broader context of learned debate.

A recurrent concern among many of these writers is the difficulty of reconciling classical notions of chance, fortune and accident with the Christian doctrine of divine providence. Often as soon as this conflict is stated, an example is offered in order to clarify the problem or to introduce a harmonizing solution. Such a pattern emerges in Book V of Boethius' *De consolatione philosophiae*, a text that was composed in late antiquity but was enormously popular in sixteenth- and seventeenth-century England.[7] When he discusses chance and fortune in this text, Boethius echoes two examples from Aristotle: the man who tills the ground and finds treasure and the unexpected encounter of two ships. The first example is used to define the concept of chance, while the second does the work of harmonization. We begin with the narrator's curious inquiry about chance and fortune as it appears in an English translation of this book published in 1609:

> "What then," quoth I, "is there nothing that can rightly bee called chance, or fortune? Or is there something, though unknowen to the common sort, to which these names agree?"
>
> "My Aristotle," quoth shee, "in his bookes of nature declared this point briefely and truely."
>
> "How?" quoth I.
>
> "When," quoth shee, "any thing is done for some certain cause, and some other thing hapneth, for some reasons than that which was intended, this is called chance: as if one digging his ground with intention to till it, findeth an

hidden treasure. This is thought to have fallen thus out by fortune, but it is not of nothing, for it hath peculiar causes, whose unexpected and not foreseene concourse seemeth to have brought forth a chance. For unlesse the Husbandman had digged up his grounds and unlesse the other had hidden his money in that place, the treasure had not been found. These are therefore the causes of this fortunate accident, which proceedeth from the meeting and concourse of causes, and not from the intention of the doer.... Wherefore wee may define chance thus: that it is an unexpected event of concurring causes [*ex confluentibus causis*] in those things which are done to some end and purpose. Now the cause, why causes concurre [*concurrere*] and meete [*confluere*] so together, is that order proceeding with inevitable connexion, which descending from the fountaine of providence, disposeth all things in their places and times [*cuncta suis locis temporibusque disponit*]."[8]

The importance of meeting and concourse, implicit in Aristotle's discussion, is made explicit in this passage through the language of concurring causes.[9] But what is most significant about this use of Aristotle's example is the way in which the meeting of causes that produces the fortuitous accident becomes inevitable from the point of view of providence, which is described as flowing like a fountain. The term used here is "disposition" of places and times, a placing of elements in different positions so that some connection or confluence becomes inevitable.

Boethius develops this very un-Aristotelian idea of a providential disposition in a passage that describes the trajectory of two ships which meet. In the poem that follows this section, the Tigris and Euphrates rivers are described as starting from the same source, dividing and then reuniting downstream—"bringing together all that both their waves doe beare." An image of controlled intermingling follows:

> The ships and trees whose rootes they from the bankes doe teare
> Will meete and they their flouds will mingle and confound,
> Yet run this wand'ring course in places which are low
> And in these sliding streames a settled law remaines.
> So fortune though it seems to runne with carelesse reins
> Yet hath it certaine rule and doth in order flow.[10]

The play of causes in this image allows Boethius to retain his Aristotelian interpretation of the accident but nest it within a larger order of control. God can, like someone far enough downstream, know that ships in the individual streams will eventually meet when the rivers join up; the ships themselves do not need direct guidance. Although this disposing agency shares some of the properties that the Stoics associated with Fate—it works through connections of causes rather than causes themselves—the image seems specifically designed to preserve the autonomy of the agents implicit in both Aristotle's theory and a Christian theology of free-will.[11] God, it seems, can pinch and stretch the topography of place and time from a great height to bring people together, even if they have determined on their own to take a certain path.

Boethius' appropriation of Aristotle's example has other transformative effects as well. On the one hand, Fortune is turned into an intermediary of God's providence when she is made the personification of the Aristotelian principle of chance. Ironically, it is the goddess herself who points toward the ancient authority when she might well be expected to claim accidents as her own. She not only becomes a spokesperson for that tradition, but provides the crucial metaphors of concourse and disposition that allow for Aristotle's category of accident to be subsumed in the spatial calculus of a paternal Christian providence. But if Fortune's powers are reassigned in this scheme, so too are those of the human agents in the world. When the pair of ships in Boethius' example meet, the accidental encounter is doubly determined, first by the pilots who steer the crafts, but then by the divinity who creates a world in which the Tigris and Euphrates meet. Accident acquires the necessity of a geographic fact, and humans are given powers of self-determination in a world that can nevertheless absorb their independent actions into a larger divine plan. This mode of providential knowledge and control is not the same kind of "doing" which was once associated with Fortune. God knows and foresees accidental events without making them happen, just as the spectator at a chariot race does not immediately cause the team out in front finally to win the match.

Aware perhaps that this kind of argument was enjoying a broad appeal in the sixteenth century, Calvin would echo Boethius' river example only to dismiss it. God is "not a mere general principle of confused motion," he writes in the *Institutes*, "as if he should command a river to flow through the channels once made for it, but a power constantly exerted on every distinct and particular movement."[12] For Calvin, the image of providence flowing through riverbeds suggests a lazy God, one who relies on general rules or preordained processes in order to accomplish his specific ends. Disposition of places and times is not enough: God needs to be actively managing those particulars as well.[13] This activism was crucial to grasp in accidental events, Calvin argued, since their hidden causes might easily suggest to the "carnal" sense that the world is governed by a blind, impetuous goddess. Usually providence is conspicuous,

> yet sometimes the causes of events are concealed, so that a suspicion intrudes itself, that the revolutions of human affairs are conducted by the blind impetuosity of fortune, or the flesh solicits us to murmur, as though God amused himself with tossing men about like tennis balls.[14]

The farcical image of tennis balls could itself be added to the catalogue of examples of accidents: like the falling statue in Aristotle's example, the balls fly about indifferently once they have been delivered into the general laws of motion. Such a comic description of divine neglect undercuts the autonomy granted to Boethius' ships sailing down independent streams and, by extension, to all of the independently acting *per se* causes that the Scholastic tradition embraced. On some level, Calvin seems to be saying that any amount of autonomy given to natural causes such as the will or nature will lead to the revival of Fortune: she has dominion only to the degree that independent, self-sustaining causes have a place in the world.

When the example of an unexpected meeting at sea metamorphoses into that of the two ships floating down the Tigris and Euphrates, Aristotle's theory gets absorbed into the dispositional account of providence. This act of appropriation allows for continuity with the classical philosophical tradition, but it also creates a liability (the passive God) that Calvin will seek to expose by redeploying the example in another direction.[15] Whether or not each reiteration in this series is a self-conscious "borrowing," the arguments and examples offered by Aristotle, Boethius and Calvin ought to be grouped together because they articulate a divergent set of possibilities inherent in a common set of examples. Calvin may not have been thinking about the Tigris and Euphrates when he made his remark about the riverbeds, and Boethius was almost certainly not thinking about tennis balls when he wrote about the providential disposition of times and places. The type of argument each wants to make, however, requires an example that is capable of restating an older position but also allows a new position to emerge. Many of Aristotle's examples possess this kind of flexibility, which is why they return again and again in arguments that begin from incompatible premises.

If the "crossing of ships" example serves as a starting point for arguments about providence, the case of unexpected meetings of people—for Aristotle, the man who goes to the market to buy something and there encounters a debtor—articulates a more eclectic set of concerns. Several such examples appear in Cicero's rhetorical treatise *Topica,* a text that served as a cornerstone of rhetorical and logical education throughout the Middle Ages.[16] The first example involves two people who meet and fall in love. If, as a result of this meeting, one member of the couple kills someone—and here Cicero relies on his reader to make the connection between love and murder—then it is improper to blame the crime on their initial meeting, which was not sufficient to bring it about.[17] The example is uncomplicated enough, reiterating Aristotle's point that not everything that happens prior to an event can be labeled a cause. Cicero makes a more interesting observation about unexpected meetings later, however, when he is focusing on the evidentiary value of such encounters rather than their causal antecedents:

> The concurrence [*concursio*] of fortuitous events [*fortuitorum*] is illustrated, for example, by a chance [*casu*] interruption when something was being said or done which should be kept secret.... Sometimes truth itself can scarcely refute evidence of this sort. (440–41)

In the context of a criminal inquiry, an unexpected encounter becomes the occasion for discovery of secrets that would otherwise remain hidden. Precisely because the interrupted party could not have anticipated the meeting, it appears that whatever he or she was doing when the meeting occurred could not have been contrived for the purposes of deception. Like the inartificial proofs mentioned in Aristotle's *Rhetoric* which compel assent without any rhetorical elaboration—signed contracts or evidence given under torture—Cicero seems to be suggesting that the accidental interruption produces evidence that automatically persuades.[18] This fascinating observation does not have a parallel in Aristotle's discussion, which focuses on the causes of accidental events rather than their effect on observers.

A powerful early modern instance of this "evidentiary principle" can be found in Shakespeare's *Othello,* a play that stages a quasi-judicial trial for infidelity around evidence which appears to have been gathered spontaneously. In the third act of the play, for example, Cassio visits Desdemona to plead his case for reconciliation with her husband after he has been stripped of his lieutenancy. As Desdemona is promising Cassio to take up his case, Iago and Othello arrive on stage just as Cassio begins to take his leave. In a brilliant display of improvisation, Iago suddenly declares, "Ha, I like not that" (3.2.33), and in doing seizes the opportunity to create suspicion about their relationship. Desdemona's trial for adultery might be said to begin at that moment, when her "guilty" conference has been unexpectedly interrupted.[19] Othello will carefully be led to believe that she is deliberately hiding something so that when she does eventually declare her innocence, her protestation will be discounted as female trickery. This skeptical tendency to trust only what is revealed involuntarily becomes an evidentiary rule of sorts as Othello is variously impressed, first by evidence reportedly given by Cassio in his sleep (3.3.423–30), and then by the handkerchief whose matter-of-fact absence is—"with the other proofs"—sufficient to decide Desdemona's guilt. Cicero's remark above about accidental discovery provides a chilling gloss on the tragedy as a whole: "Sometimes the truth itself can scarcely refute evidence of this sort."

While Cicero and Shakespeare use the accidental meeting of persons to suggest that unexpected events are a crooked (and unreliable) path of discovery in a world of deceit, the example of the accidental meeting does a very different kind of work in the theological texts of Albertus Magnus and those of his student, Thomas Aquinas. Both of these writers are direct inheritors of Aristotle's distinctions and examples via the *Physics*; each, moreover, is aware of the problems that arise when one accepts Aristotle's definition of the accidental efficient causes of chance or fortune without qualification. Albert gives a characteristically exhaustive survey of the problems before testing one of the solutions with an example. On the face of it, Albert writes in his commentary on the *Physics*, chance or fortuitous events are an affront to the church's teaching on God's providence.[20] Several have tried to solve this problem by invoking alternate means of control: for example, the astrologers or *Mathematici* posit a stellar necessity that governs accidental events from above.[21] Yet even stellar influence working as an instrument of divine providence is not decisive in such cases, Albert argues elsewhere, and so the belief in chance and fortune would seem to be "quasi-contradictory."[22] Such a belief implies both that such events are inexorable (that is, they "must happen" because God foresees them) and yet still contingent (they "may or may not" happen depending on the circumstances).

Once the contradiction has been stated, Albert is ready to introduce the example of an unexpected meeting, one that echoes Aristotle's example about the meeting in the marketplace but adds another level of necessary causation. Some who have tried to integrate accidents with the doctrine of divine control, he writes, have said that everything which happens must be compared to both its particular and universal causes, the latter being the order of the motion of the heavens [*ordo motus caelestium*] or the first cause, which is God. Those who think this way argue that chance and fortune are real with respect to particular causes, since many things happen outside the intention [*praeter intentionem*] of those causes, yet are necessary with respect to God. To explain their views, they use a simile:

> There is a rich master with many slaves who—unknown to them—also has some sheep that have fallen into a trap; he wants his slaves to save the sheep when they discover them. He tells the slaves to go to the place where the trap is, into which the animals have fallen, and does not tell the slaves why they go there, nor does he tell one that the other is going there, but tells them separately to go to the place by different ways. Of these slaves, one does not expect to discover the other next to the pit, nor does the other expect to rescue the animals from the pit, because they do not know that the animals had fallen into the pit. And for this reason the animals are rescued and saved from the pit by chance according to the slaves, and by chance they discover each other next to the pit, and nevertheless for the master none of these things happens by chance.[23]

The added armature of the master who sets up the meeting, of course, allows the unexpected encounter from Aristotle to serve a vastly different argumentative purpose. While the meeting is clearly unexpected to those involved, it is no accident if Albert is using Aristotle's definition of the term, since the two slaves are instruments of the master's will instead of truly independent agents. The reason why some have found the example appealing, Albert suggests, is that it eliminates what is accidental about such meetings without dismissing the individual's experience of some events as having no discernible *per se* cause.

But there is a difficulty involved in placing this deliberate narrative shell around the original accident: just as it is intended to do, the modification delivers control over the "accident" to the mind of the master—in this case, God. Albert points out that if one accepts this addition to the story, chance and fortune do indeed disappear, but so do free will and deliberation.[24] In order to avoid this crucial loss, Albert argues that one must adopt Aristotle's notion of accidental causes and understand that God can foresee accidents even though they have no *per se* causes. While it is not fully worked out in this passage, Albert is moving toward an elegant solution, since by asserting the real contingency of sublunar events he can credit human choice to agents other than God without making God ignorant of those choices.[25] The challenge, however, will be to give a more detailed explanation of how God knows these events which manifestly lack any metaphysical necessity that would allow them to be foreseen.

Taking up the example of the unexpected meeting of slaves once again, Thomas Aquinas (1225–74) provides just this kind of explanation. In Aquinas's hands, the contrived "accidental" meeting becomes significant as a demonstration that such encounters are ultimately grasped in a mental space; in doing so he subtly shifts the starting point for understanding providential accidents from a divine perspective to a human one. Immediately following his defense of the existence of accidental events in his commentary on Aristotle's *De interpretatione*, Aquinas turns to the role of the mind in unifying the dispersed causes of accidents:

> However, we must now note that the merely incidental can be apprehended as a unity by mind: being white and being a musician, which in themselves are two things not one, can be taken as one by a mind framing a single proposition connecting them. And this is the way it can sometimes happen that an event which in itself happens incidentally and by chance can be traced back to a mind that has set it up beforehand: as the meeting of two slaves in a certain place—which as far as they are concerned is incidental and chance because they didn't know about each other—can nevertheless have been intended by their master.[26]

The example from Albert's commentary is used here to demonstrate the way in which the mind can comprehend, and thus even premeditate, the connection between two things that are not intrinsically connected. Just as a mind can grasp that the property of whiteness occurs accidentally in a substance (John) that is musical, so too, Aquinas is arguing in this extended analogy, the mind can grasp the accidental meeting of two individuals as a unity and sometimes even make such a meeting happen. The analogy is not a very good one, however, since the master who sets up the meeting of the slaves really supplies their meeting with a unitary cause of a kind that is missing in the case of the white musician. The assumption that a particular category of human being can become the instrument of another—essential to the analogy—is, moreover, at odds with Scholastic doctrine on the fundamental independence of the human will.

If the example of a "contrived" meeting of slaves creates as many problems as it solves, why does Aquinas use it? He seems to be drawn to the example because, for at least a moment, it allows him to isolate an associative brand of human knowledge which can serve as the pattern for God's nonnecessitating knowledge of accidental events. Once this capacity for association is understood, the coercive act in which God actually commands that accidents happen can be postponed or perhaps even abandoned.[27] An entire epistemology of both accidents and divine foresight will have to be offered if the problematic aspects of the example are to be eliminated, something that Aquinas does in his discussion of God's knowledge in the *Summa theologiae*. The outlines of that theory are worth rehearsing here, since it prepares the way for a hypothetical return to Aristotle's example in its original form.

As humans, Aquinas writes, we can have knowledge of what is happening at present, memory of what has happened in the past, and "foreknowledge" of what will happen in the future based on our grasp of secondary causes.[28] We do not foresee accidents, then, because these events do not have the kind of regular causes from which we could predict them. We can, however, see accidental unities in the present. For example, I can see that John is sitting in front of me right now and so have knowledge of the connection of this accidental predicate—sitting—with a particular substance, John. The sitting thing and John are not, however, the same thing in any metaphysical sense. The seated John is an accidental unity, "one" in a less-than-metaphysical sense that we can know by sight or report but never deduce or predict. (Contemporary readers of Aristotle still argue about the nature of this kind of unity of substance and accident, calling it a "kooky object"—a term that has not yet been applied to accidental events.)[29]

Aquinas asks his reader to compare this kind of human knowledge with God's knowledge and foresight of accidental events. Unlike us, Aquinas writes in his commentary on *De interpretatione*, God sees all events in time as one eternal present. Factual propositions that he knows are not qualified by tense:

So in his one glance he sees everything going on throughout time, and each as it is in itself, not as something future to himself and his seeing and visible only as it exists within its causal situation (although he sees that causal situation). But he sees things altogether eternally, each as it exists in its own time, just as our own human eye sees John sitting there himself, not just as something determined by causes. Nor does our seeing John sitting there stop it being an event that might not have been when regarded just in relation to its causes. And yet while he is sitting there we see him sitting there with certainty and without doubt, since when a thing exists in itself it is already determined. In this way then God knows everything that happens in time with certainty and without doubt, and yet the things that happen in time are not things that must exist or must come to exist, but things that might or might not be.[30]

Although the accident is not metaphysically necessary, nor even probable, it can be grasped outside of its determining causes as a "certain" fact in the present by sight. Aquinas has isolated the particularly visual character of this kind of knowledge, the way in which to know the accident is almost the same as to see it.[31] The blind necessity of an accident is thus like that blank facticity that attends a thing's sitting there in front of us, but of course we—limited by the time in which we may look and the places we can see—can gain that knowledge only in the present or remember it from the past. The ideal vantage point, here the fantastic position occupied by an eternal being, offers certain knowledge of future events that have no intrinsic causes, a position which resembles that of a theatrical spectator who, seeing a play for the second time, knows what will happen before it actually comes to pass. Aquinas's epistemology of accident thus clears the way for Aristotle's original example of an accidental meeting in the marketplace to be embraced without modification: if God has a tenseless knowledge of the present, there is no obstacle to his foreseeing that the debtor will accidentally meet his lender tomorrow, just as there is no obstacle to his foreseeing the contingent choice of each to enter the market on a particular day.

A final example of this type, this one from Nicole Oresme's *De causis mirabilium,* demonstrates how the accidental meeting of people can be used to dampen speculation on the supernatural causes of unusual events—one of the major themes of this fourteenth-century treatise on the causes of marvels.[32] In the course of his discussion, Oresme introduces the example of a man named Sortes (which is the Latin word for "chance") who has just stolen a horse. After he has committed the crime, Sortes encounters a maniac on the street who announces: "You have just stolen a horse." Such an event is marvelous, but it does not necessarily demonstrate that the maniac has extraordinary powers of perception. While there may be a subtle causal principle at work here, Oresme writes, it also is possible that the maniac is just speaking something which by chance [*casu*] happened to be true. The example is significant because it suggests that the dramatic force of both the meeting and the maniac's subsequent announcement can be dampened by viewing the event as a strictly natural occurrence with no causal significance. The example of accidental truth-telling also "doubles" the accidental meeting of persons on another, figurative level, since it implies a "meeting" of communicative contexts that overlap and so produce wonder and confusion. (This type of overlap is the basis for the plot of Shakespeare's *Comedy of Errors,* the subject of the next chapter.) To the extent that this overlap is not deliberate but coincidental, the maniac's utterance seems to serve a purpose that he could not have intended: meaning as well as meeting are accidental in this example.

Elsewhere in *De causis mirabilium,* Oresme takes up the question of monsters and monstrous births—a third type of exemplary accident derived from Aristotle that we can trace into the early modern period. Already the subject of contentious philosophical debates in the fourteenth century when Oresme was writing his treatise, monstrous births became a sociopolitical concern as laypersons and priests took liberties in attributing divine or demonic agency to anomalous phenomena.[33] Why would God do such things directly by miraculous intervention or assign the work of marvel-making to demons, Oresme asks, when he could just as easily work through causes that are well known? Oresme's reluctance to embrace the extravagant answer leads him to affirm the role of chance in the production of monsters rather than some extraordinary plastic power working directly in the womb, a version of which had already been affirmed by Albert and the astrologers. Sensitive to the diversity of causes in the world and the variable conditions in which they must work, Oresme describes the process of generation as the scene of an encounter: a variety of conditions and agents must meet in the proper manner for development to be successful.[34] We should not marvel then when the process goes awry, he writes, just as we should not marvel when a heated piece of lead is thrown to the ground and by chance [*forte*] takes the shape of a man or a bird.

The example of lead "falling" into an unusual shape is effective because it analogizes an unobservable accidental deviation in generation to a visible process of falling—one that is reminiscent of Aristotle's example of a falling tripod which happens to land on its feet. Like the paint spatterings that would fascinate Italian Renaissance artists in search of creative inspiration, the monstrous birth is like an image made by chance—a spontaneous production which only accidentally resembles some other kind of creature (or perhaps even a type of human), and so cannot be explained on the basis of that similarity. Oresme's impulse to give a physical example of the experientially remote mechanism of accidental generation is not unique. Aquinas, for example, when describing the causes of a six-fingered baby in the *Summa contra gentiles*, goes to a familiar topos from Aristotle to clarify his position: the child is produced by an intermingling of independent causal processes, an explanation that recalls the intersecting paths of causal agents in the *Metaphysics*.[35] Albert too will use an Aristotelian conception of accident to explain the source of monstrous births, recognizing that at times "something in the works of nature happens outside the intention of nature, such as a sixth finger, or two heads on one body, or the absence of a finger."[36] Here the purposiveness of natural processes assumed in Aristotle's example is amplified as nature rather than God becomes an artificer whose intentions are subject to unforeseen alterations. For Albert at least, there is something to be gained by making "errors of nature," or *pecatta naturae,* the result of an accidental crossing of causal lines: the divinely ordained regularity of nature is preserved and God is relieved of immediate responsibility for deviations.

In the early modern period, the monster becomes a powerful example of the creativity of nature and the immediacy of God's judgment on human affairs; it also serves as an occasion for the same kind of naturalistic explanation that Oresme advocated in the fourteenth century. In the works of Pierre Boaistuau and Conrad Lycosthenes, for example, monsters could be viewed as both natural and portentous at the same time, making them paradigm for the cooperation of divine and secondary causes in the sixteenth and seventeenth centuries.[37] The possibility of viewing monsters as the result of chance or some other natural cause—for example the maternal imagination, emanations from the stars, the defects of matter—did not, however, mean that early modern writers were always ready to provide both natural and supernatural forms of explanation at the same time. Francis Bacon, for example, focused primarily on monsters as natural particulars or anomalies in order to correct hasty generalizations about their causal antecedents.[38] Martin Luther, on the other hand, would be emphatic in pointing out the divine meaning of such events, for example in his 1523 pamphlet written with Philipp Melanchthon on the "Pope-ass" and the "monk-calf"—monstrous births that were thought to signify God's displeasure with monastic corruption.[39]

The example of the monster produced by accident persisted in learned and popular texts in the sixteenth and seventeenth centuries with its Aristotelian pedigree intact. The pseudo-Aristotelian *Problemata*, for example, pointed out a variety of ways in which the process of generation could misfire, and the French surgeon Ambroise Paré was sympathetic to the Aristotelian analysis of monsters (among others) in his *Des Monstres et prodiges*.[40] Regardless of its persistence as an explanatory category, however, accident would not prove conclusive as a means of emptying monsters and other "preternatural" phenomena of their supernatural meaning. Oresme was wrong to assume that marvelous anomalies would be less appealing to the religious interpreter when they were shown to result from a coincidence or convergence. Accident and divine signification are incompatible only if accidental divergences are understood in the strictly Aristotelian sense as having no cause whatsoever. To the extent that an unusual production in the womb—or indeed, any anomalous phenomenon in the world—was understood to involve a rare meeting of causal lines, it would always be possible to ask why those lines came to cross in this particular place and at this particular time. Was God really forbidden to arrange such meetings? Such questions were put most forcefully by Jean Calvin in his reappraisal of God's providential action. Here the fourth and final accident type, the errant or falling object, becomes an emblem for the power of creation to continue on its own divinely ordained course, regardless of human wants or desires.

Catastrophes involving errant or falling objects conjure up pagan notions of chance and fortune for Calvin, which is perhaps why he regularly uses them as examples in the *Institutes.* Like the man who might be killed by a falling roof tile in the quotation at the beginning of this chapter, the individual in Calvin's providential world may suddenly be "taken" from above, an event that appears at first to be an unfortunate accident, but which should ultimately be understood as a deliberate act:

> Scripture, more fully to express that nothing is transacted in the world but according to his destination, shows that those things are subject to him which appear most fortuitous. For what would you be more ready to attribute to chance, than when a limb broken off from a tree kills a passing traveller? But very different is the decision of the Lord, who acknowledges that he has delivered him into the hand of the slayer.[41]

The example of the falling branch is effective because, unlike a person, the branch is not capable of altering its own direction. When Calvin uses such an example, he is inviting readers to adopt the view of the universe which holds that objects in the world simply combine out of an indifferent necessity. Such a view is useful to invoke temporarily, since it foregrounds the drama of the example. Like purposes fallen upon their inventors' heads, the indifference of bodies in motion to their destination gives them an almost unique power to mark out the unmovable limits to human agency.

What is most significant about such examples for Calvin, however—and here he is introducing an idea that will resonate far into the seventeenth century—is that they activate a saving knowledge of God's presence and direction in the world, part of the "knowledge of God" that is one of the two major themes of the *Institutes.*[42] Such a knowledge, Calvin argues, is naturally present in the mind and continually refreshed by our encounters with creation: it is this experiential or "experimental" component of our engagement with providence, understood as an encounter with human frailty and dependence on God, which Calvin believes will lead the individual to faith.[43] In an almost anthropological moment of speculation, Calvin makes this nascent knowledge of providence a universal attribute of humanity, even where scriptural revelation is lacking. The "Philistine

Sorcerers," for example, "though they fluctuated in uncertainty, ascribed adverse accidents partly to God, partly to fortune."[44] Such a willingness to contemplate God as a cause of their suffering is, for Calvin, a testimony to the fact that "the Scriptural doctrine of special providence has never been totally removed from the hearts of men." In setting out vivid examples of accidental events throughout the *Institutes,* Calvin is engaging that untutored consciousness of God's providence and attempting to shape it into a coherent form of devotion.[45]

Other writers in the learned tradition had invoked similar accidents to illustrate the palpable indifference of natural processes (such as falling or motion) to deliberate human manipulation, but unlike Calvin these writers severed the link between reflection on such occasions and the acquisition of knowledge. When, for example, Cicero points out in his *Topica* that it is possible to exonerate the accused by showing how his weapon struck a blow by chance, the argument for innocence rests on the assumption that what happens by chance or accident cannot be known in advance. When faced with such an example, auditors are expected to relinquish any further interest in the cause of the outcome—how, after all, can the causes of such accidents be practically known?—and absolve the doer of the deed. So too, when Boethius describes a rock falling on the head of a man who has gone to visit a friend, or Aquinas mentions a fiery body that has fallen to earth in precisely the place where something combustible lies, each assumes that the manifest indifference of projectiles to their destinations will empty the accident of any knowable cause.[46] In such a world in which things are assumed to meet and combine blindly, humans are without advance knowledge of accidents: these events are not yet instances that will testify to God's active presence in the world, as they will be for Calvin and his English interpreters. Instead, they stand at the *ne plus ultra* of human knowledge and foresight, a threshold that Bacon will attempt to breach with his reforms in natural philosophy.

Like the other accidents surveyed in this chapter, the career of the errant or falling object illustrates how radically different conclusions can be attached to a core set of examples. The Scholastic reluctance to see a hidden cause behind the accident seems almost intuitive when Albert invokes the example of the tripod falling in the position of a seat. But when Calvin describes a branch falling on a passing traveler's head, or a single step committing the sea traveler to certain death, the experience of contingency—which is to say, the realization that circumstances could easily have been otherwise—leads the surprised or baffled individual in a different direction. For Calvin and others who saw accidents as proofs of God's abiding creativity and interest, these events could not be resigned to the intellectual void created for them by Aristotle and his Scholastic interpreters: instead they needed to be recognized as a means for apprehending and so knowing God's designing presence in the world. Under the auspices of special providence, the unexpected would soon become a source of spiritual knowledge during the late sixteenth century, even if philosophical knowledge of the unexpected was too much to ask.[47]

But while God's presence might be known through accidents, the specific character of his wishes and judgments was difficult if not impossible to grasp in Calvin's scheme. In a fascinating passage about the difficulty of understanding providential judgments, Calvin writes that the Psalmist, once he has described several "wonderful" examples of divine succor, such as bringing the shipwrecked into port,

> infers from them that what are accounted fortuitous accidents, are so many proofs of his heavenly providence, especially of his paternal clemency.... But, since the majority of men, immersed in their errors, are blind amidst the greatest opportunities of seeing [Fr. *ne voit gutte en un si beau theatre*; L. *in tam illustri theatro caecutit*], he accounts it a rare instance of singular wisdom discreetly to consider these works of God; from the sight of which, some, who, in other instances, discover the greatest acuteness, receive no benefit.[48]

Calvin's sense that the world is a place of spectacle and that accidents are perhaps the most wondrous and bewildering instances of his pervasive control would be reiterated by English religious writers who were much more aggressive about identifying God's providential designs in accidental events. In Calvin's view, it is quite rare that an individual can really understand God's secret counsels in such events. Instead of curiosity, he recommends an Augustinian awe at creation as a whole, "fainting, as it were, under [God's] immensity, we must take a view of his works, that we may be refreshed with his goodness."[49] Scripture urges us, he writes, to attend to this "magnificent theater ... which is replete with innumerable miracles ...

from the contemplation of which we ought wisely to acquire the knowledge of God."[50]

But Calvin also senses a certain dramatic irony in God's providential works. To demonstrate his power, God often takes the wise "in their own craftiness" or forces them to "fall by their own exertions," waiting for the best possible "occasion" on which to make his point.[51] By making a deliberate effort to "dispose" and arrange agents in such a way as to impress the human spectator, Calvin's God becomes the governing force in a world that is structured along the lines of a theater. To the extent that individuals are alive to the poetics of that theater, they may wonder endlessly at the immense scope and power of providence, even if they are forbidden from knowing exactly what God means to do at a particular time and place. Such knowledge of the "how" and "why" of providence is ultimately less important for Calvin than the knowledge "that" God is at work in the world. The latter kind of knowledge is to be had in the theater of the world—a place of beholding where accidents imply for spectators that some guiding force has contrived events for a reason.

Like an errant weapon, Calvin suggests, the plots and devices of individuals will return to do them harm, highlighting for worldly spectators the theatrical nature of their own experience. As the common instrument of tragic downfall and divine punishment, the falling object is an appropriate figure with which to end this survey of Aristotelian accident types, since it suggests an important convergence to come. In the next century, as English writers such as Phillip Stubbes, Thomas Field and the translator Thomas Beard begin chronicling striking accidents in the world, the cousin realms of world and stage will be linked together in a dense network of analogies and providential narratives. Such narratives will regularly gloss accidents as tragic, wondrous or awe inspiring, precisely the powers that Aristotle seemed to reserve for them as a device of the theater. In the work of Calvin, we find articulated the underlying set of assumptions that makes those narratives and analogies possible—not simply as a common poetic intuition—but a comprehensive theory of experience. At the center of that theory was God, and at the periphery, a spectator who might suddenly awaken to a knowledge of that God's presence at the moment when experience seemed as spontaneous as it was contrived.

CHAPTER 3

The Avoidance of Ends in 'The Comedy of Errors'

> *E. Antipholus*: To what end did I bid thee hie thee home?
> *E. Dromio*: To a rope's end, sir, and to that end am I returned.
> *E. Antipholus*: And to that end, sir, I will welcome you.
> [Beats Dromio] (4.4.15–18)

Since its notorious performance at the Gray's Inn revels in 1594, *The Comedy of Errors* has had a curious relationship to accidental events. When the play was presented on the evening of December 28, the crowd was so large that it could not be accommodated in the hall, a minor catastrophe of sorts since the resulting confusion delayed presentation of the play and forced many spectators to leave early. One witness described the affair as a "mischanceful Accident," a scene so chaotic that some of those present in the audience were later put on mock trial by the pretend "Prince" of the revels and his "Lawyers" for using "Sorceries," "Enchantments," "vain Representations and shews" to incite the crowd to disorder.[1] Like the errors in the play itself, the confusion at Gray's Inn was eventually dismissed as harmless, comic mischance rather than the work of some "Sorcerer or Conjurer." The "trial" that followed the casualties of this first performance suggests that those who managed actually to see the play that night were sensitive to some of its most intriguing questions: how does one represent an accident without suggesting that it serves some deliberate purpose or diabolical end? Is there any way to stop the suspicious mind once it has been set in motion, or will inquiry into "disorder" only slow down when a hidden purpose is found, preferably in some guilty mind, toward which all events have been tending?

In the play, of course, those who think they are being gulled or abused eventually relinquish their suspicions when they see that a specific set of circumstances (rather than some malicious agent) is responsible for the confusion on stage. Accusations of theft, infidelity, and insubordination vanish when characters recognize that two sets of identical twins have met "accidentally" in the city streets of Ephesus and—failing to recognize this fact—have repeatedly mistaken one another in a process of coordinated or "sympathizèd" error. Because the plot pivots on a sequence of hapless exchanges in which this accident fails to be discovered, *The Comedy of Errors* is often singled out among Shakespeare's plays as emotionally superficial or metaphysically vacuous. Harold Jenkins, for example, is critical of the play because "the confusion is really the result of accidental circumstances and is as accidentally cleared up."[2] While Jenkins and others may have been too quick to dismiss the play as "mere farce," they have a point. More than any other play in the Shakespearean canon, *The Comedy of Errors* relies on accidental events to defer and then bring about comic resolution. The play's conclusion seems almost perfectly indifferent to the deliberate action of any of its characters, a feature that has prompted critics to see the shuffle on stage as arbitrary, mechanical, even inhumane.[3]

Yet *The Comedy of Errors* is more than a story about the perils of supposition in a world of coincidence, even if the bizarre premise of two sets of identical twins seems to authorize this interpretation. While it is clearly an outrageous farce, the play is also a precise and quite relentless analysis of the nature of accidental events and the rhetorical means by which they are grasped or misunderstood in social situations. Such a "trial by farce" reveals something that the shorter examples from the philosophical texts discussed earlier could only hint at: that narratives about accidents, precisely because they are narratives, will suggest some deeper purpose or "end" which accidents serve, regardless of whether or not that purpose actually exists. The play can thus be read as a theatrical fable about the avoidance of ends, both in the sense of narrative endings and the purposes that get attached to accidental events in specific situations. When read in these terms, *The Comedy of Errors* explores a number of interlocking philosophical and rhetorical problems that a more analytic text could only gesture at. Foremost among these is the difficulty of representing accidents as such, a difficulty that is as much a function of the unusual rhetorical situations in which accidents must be described as it is of the philosophical opacity of accidents themselves.

Coleridge, when comparing this play with other comedies, remarked that *The Comedy of Errors* is "the only poetical farce" in English, suggesting that as a species of drama Shakespeare's play is as odd as the events it portrays. In discussing the license taken in the plot, he clarifies an aspect of the play's excess which is crucial to its farcical mode of trial and demonstration:

A proper farce is mainly distinguished from comedy by the license allowed, and even required, in the fable, in order to produce strange and laughable situations. The story need not be probable, it is enough that it is possible. A comedy would scarcely allow even the two Antipholuses; because, although there have been instances of almost indistinguishable likeness in two persons, yet these are mere individual accidents, *casus ludentis naturae*, and the *verum* will not excuse the *inverisimile*.[4]

Not only does the plot test the limits of theatrical "belief" as to how many accidents might be possible, but the twins themselves seem a chance of playing nature. The singularity of these conditions—what we might call the extravagance of chance manifested in the two sets of twins and their chiasmatic criss-crossings—is precisely what gives the play its force as an extended philosophical example. Leaving aside for the moment the question of what is demonstrated by such an example, we should recognize that Coleridge situates the farcical accident in the category of the true but nonetheless extremely unlikely. Like twins or other deviations from the usual course of nature, accidents prove that what is true-to-life in art is bound by conventions that nature sometimes does not honor. But what is accepted in nature cannot be excused in the artist, and it is for this imposition of improbable "accidents" on the verisimilar world of a dramatic work of art that Shakespeare's play is often censured.

Like many other aesthetic categories, verisimilitude is a convention that is honored as much in the breach as it is in the observance. Within comedy, accidents have regularly functioned in ways that seem arbitrary or improbable.[5] Many of Shakespeare's early comedies, for example, rely on unpurposed events to bring about important dramatic changes, but have fared somewhat better against charges of excess. The confusion in *Love's Labour's Lost*, for example, which follows when Berowne's letter to Rosaline is "accidentally, or by way of progression . . . miscarried" to Jaquenetta, is dramatically indispensable (4.2.137–38). Meetings of specific characters that are not intended by anyone on stage are also important to some of these early plays. Vincentio, for example, is "happily" met by Petruchio and Kate in the forest (4.5) and then surprises his impersonator in act five of *The Taming of the Shrew*. Valentine stumbles into an ambush in the forest (4.1), precipitating his alliance with the outlaws, which, in turn, allows him to capitalize on the capture of the other lovers in the final scene of *The Two Gentlemen of Verona*.[6]

Several of these early plays rely on accident to bring about important transitions, yet none is as deliberate as *The Comedy of Errors* in using such events as a structural device for creating comic effects. The arbitrary premise of two pairs of twins, their accidental separation and their coincidental meeting in Ephesus, make it absolutely clear to the audience that the errors are not devised by any "practicer" on stage, nor necessitated by any predictable natural process.[7] It is on this presumption that spectators can identify a "gap in understanding" or laughable mismatch between the repeated complaint of the characters—that they are being gulled, abused, or led astray on purpose—and the fact that no such motivation, cause, or end can be seen to exist.[8] Characters are thus plagued not simply by their confusion in the face of unexpected events but also by their understanding of them, so much so that error itself has become synonymous with intuition or comprehension. More important, accident and coincidence have become the means by which that human capacity for erroneous understanding gets broken down into its situational—and as I will argue, rhetorical—components. Given the stated desire of Francis Bacon (who also wrote something for the Gray's Inn revels of 1594) to rid natural philosophy of its sources of error or "Idols," the intellectual stakes in a farce like *The Comedy of Errors* are potentially quite high.[9] In providing a concrete set of situations in which error can be assayed, the play is more than a dramatic diversion or an exercise in a young playwright's command of plotting. It is an engine for inquiry.

Error in this play works like an inflating bubble which grows whenever anyone tries to offer a narrative account of his or her dealings with other characters. This dynamic of rhetorical "inflation" takes hold because the simple act of putting one's confusion into words is, ironically, the very means by which the accidental source of error is made more difficult to recognize. One gets the sense—plainly articulated by the Dromios, who are regularly beaten for what they say—that every time someone opens his or her mouth, things can only get worse. And indeed, things do get worse as characters are variously beaten, mocked, exorcised, arrested or otherwise abused. What is amazing about this situation is that the mayhem is sustained for such a long time.[10] Part of what sustains this confusion, as I have already suggested, is not just the fact that a single pair of twins never manages to meet until act five. The play also avoids its ending every time a character tells a story about what has happened.

The Duke is the one who articulates the way in which accidents and their narrative representation have sustained the confusion throughout. When Emilia begins to recognize herself in Egeon's tale, the Duke tells the audience in an aside:

> Why, here begins his morning story right:
> These two Antipholus', these two so like,
> And these two Dromios, one in semblance—
> Besides his urging of her wrack at sea.
> These are the parents to these children,
> Which accidentally are met together. (5.1.348–53)

At the conclusion of the play we are given, through the Duke's eyes, a vision of a story set right, one in which servants and masters are correctly understood to have met accidentally in the Ephesian market. The Duke's use of the term "story" is crucial, since it emphasizes the way in which the comic ending is as much a harmonization of narratives as it is a readjustment of social identities and a sorting out of bodies.[11]

While the Duke's final aside points out the difficulty of matching different narratives in the play—narratives that make up more than a third of the text[12]—it also encourages us to understand the play as a whole as one long attempt to give a narrative account of accidents as such. To the extent that the rhetorical mode of these stories sustains and comments on that effort, we can begin to grasp the way in which these modes serve as an index of the play's stalled progress toward the final resolution in act five. I want now to examine several scenes of narrative recapitulation to see how they contribute to or comment upon this broader problem of representing accidents in a purpose-neutral way. I will begin with the long story Egeon tells about his past in the opening scene, moving forward with the flow of the plot to examine several short descriptions of past action in acts two through four. Several other narratives—the two opposed pleas of Adriana and her husband before the Duke and the story that the Duke will hear "at large discoursed" in the Abbey—will broaden out the analysis before I conclude with a discussion of the play itself as an accident narrative, one that attempts to avoid the same sources of misunderstanding it dramatizes on stage.

Egeon's self-conscious narrative of his shipwreck is a romance tale of accidents at sea and long-lost siblings, one which suggests that everything that has happened to him is governed by an indifferent Fortune.[13] While the speech serves the dramatic function of furnishing the audience with crucial information about the twins, it also provides a detailed illustration of the way in which accidents can be rhetorically transformed into purposive actions or outcomes. He begins by disclaiming any responsibility for his troubles:

> A heavier task could not have been imposed
> Than I to speak my griefs unspeakable.
> Yet, that the world may witness that my end
> Was wrought by nature, not by vile offense,
> I'll utter what my sorrow gives me leave. (1.1.31–35)

The *aporia* here is disingenuous, since what follows is the most voluble narration of events offered in the play. Egeon's highly conventional *narratio* is a virtual catalogue of tropes for contingency, his references to his own "hap," "mishap," and his "hapless" life marking the story's progress in their constant repetition.[14] The term "hap" is not the Latinate "accident" used by the Duke but originates in early middle English, where it refers to what "falls" or "befalls" a person by chance or luck.[15] The first two lines of the play which Egeon speaks, "Proceed, Solinus, to procure my fall, / And by the doom of death end woes and all" might be read as putting this definition of hap as what "falls" into a neat couplet. Egeon's story will conceptually rhyme "all" with "fall," rendering a world—apparently the one of this play—in which hap or Fortune is the cause of all events.[16]

The story that Egeon tells suggests that his presence in Ephesus is, rather paradoxically, the "end" toward which a series of chance events led. When his factor's death in Epidamnum leaves his goods "at random," Egeon departs from Syracuse to attend to his affairs. Once there he is joined by his wife, who gives birth to twins. By coincidence, a "mean woman" happens to be staying in the same house and gives birth to another set of twins, which Egeon purchases. When they try to return home, the "tragic" winds begin to blow ominously. Just as they sight the ships that might rescue them, Egeon says:

> We were encountered by a mighty rock,
> Which being violently borne upon,
> Our helpful ship was splitted in the midst,
> So that in this unjust divorce of us
> Fortune had left to both of us alike
> What to delight in, what to sorrow for. (1.1.101–6)

The "which" of the second line above and the passive voice of the first confuse agent and patient in a way that almost empties the collision of any cause. Just as it seems the group was met by an active, personified rock, the perspective switches and the rock is "born upon" by the "helpful" but hapless "ship," which is itself "splitted." Egeon's story leaves this crucial, enabling moment of the play in a causal and rhetorical void. The lack of agent here clears the way for a more powerful one, "Fortune," which is all the more effective because its place in guiding events is left unsupplied.

If this story seems rhetorically overwrought because of its generic coding and formal narrative structure, it also shows signs of sophistication in its careful management of agency. Because the accident of the shipwreck lacks any mundane causal explanation, rhetorical convention and conceit (that is, manipulation of voice, self-conscious narrative disposition, personification) have come to compensate for that explanatory lack. The contrived quality of Egeon's speech may thus be a symptom of a deeper, philosophical difficulty. When no preceding causal nexus exists for the meeting of ship and rock, there are no explanatory constraints (if he is really aiming at an explanation) on how he narrates the event. The cause of the event becomes eminently "assignable," and rhetoric—in the sense of a form of discourse that takes explanatory priority over its content—becomes the mark of some ontological disconnect between the world and the stories that must represent it. Without a causal guardrail to limit it, narrative explanation of an accident has become a form of rhetorical wandering in this scene. The coherence that such an explanation provides, moreover, acquires the status of a quasi-manneristic conceit.

In cases in which causes are missing, agency and purpose must be supplied by the speaker, and the one that Egeon supplies is hyperbolic and somewhat perverse. After describing his shipwreck, he pauses:

> Thus have you heard me severed from my bliss,
> That by misfortunes was my life prolonged
> To tell sad stories of my own mishaps. (1.1.118–20)

Egeon's story is not simply a tale about contingency, but another one of its artifacts. Pointing to a "life prolonged to tell sad stories," he incorporates his own forlorn, speaking presence into the narrative as its destination, preposterously locating the reason for past events in the fact that he must eventually arrive in Ephesus to describe them.[17] Although Egeon's end was "wrought by nature, not by vile offense," listeners get the sense that there was some purpose guiding the winds that overrode all of his plans. Egeon has been preserved to tell stories about what has happened to him, and from his story the listener is asked to see the mere fact of his speaking as evidence that some larger force has destined him to do so.[18]

In a manner that is emblematic of the problems of narrative description which haunt the play, the coordinating conjunction plays an ambiguous role in mediating relationships between different elements in Egeon's story. The connective "and," for example, is repeatedly used to introduce accidental outcomes in Egeon's shipwreck story, dilating the sequence of events without necessarily connecting them causally. When the fishermen from Corinth discover Emilia, for example, Egeon says:

> Her part, poor soul, seeming as burdenèd
> With lesser weight but not with lesser woe,
> Was carried with more speed before the wind,
> And in our sight they three were taken up
> By fishermen of Corinth, as we thought. (1.1.107–11)

Again the use of the passive voice, along with the logical flatness of the "And" that introduces Emilia's rescuers, perfectly sidesteps any judgment on the cause of her meeting with the fishermen. We can read the causal ambiguity of the word "and" here as a grammatical illustration of a larger problem: because narrative conjunction combines two different kinds of sequence—the metonymic "and then" of narrative exposition and the "and then" of causal consequence—it embodies the unhappy merger of rhetorical and causal connection which the play suggests must eventually be separated.[19]

The conjunction also symbolizes Egeon's weary obligation to continue a story that he cannot conclude because, ultimately, it will not let him stop speaking. After he describes the shipwreck and his lost family, the Duke asks Egeon to "dilate at full / What have befall'n of them and thee till now." The story is continued with an odd mixture of conviction and listlessness: having lost one son to the storm and the other to the search for his brother, Egeon has traveled alone through Greece and Asia in search of both, only to make a fatal turn into this hostile port of Ephesus. Again, it is an "and" that introduces a crucial turn of events:

> Five summers have I spent in farthest Greece,
> Roaming clean through the bounds of Asia,
> And coasting homeward came to Ephesus (1.1.132–35)

With this last episode, Egeon coasting into the bay where he will be ransomed against death, the speaker has reached the point where the present of the story coincides with the moment at which that story is spoken. When the two meet it is time to stop. "But here must end the story of my life," Egeon avers, but he cannot resist tacking on an event which, if it were to take place, would provide a happy conclusion: "And happy were I in my timely death / Could all my travels warrant me they live" (1.1.138–39).

Egeon's last lines before the group leaves—"Hopeless and helpless doth Egeon wend, / But to procrastinate his lifeless end" (1.1.157–58)—cements the link between narrative exposition and errant wandering, a link that is articulated on the level of the play's structure. Recognizing that the play unfolds through a process of "dilation," as Patricia Parker has described it, we can say that there is always an "and" that comes to defer Egeon's "end," making it appear as if his life is literally prolonged by the story he now tells.[20] "Hopeless and helpless" also resonate with "hapless," hinting further at Egeon's equation of his own diminished prospects and his passivity toward an overwhelming power of "hap" or Fortune. From Egeon's point of view his fate is already determined, and so the only option is to embrace willfully an end to suffering in the form of death, even to desire it. There is no room for contingency in this tale of misfortune; rather, all events are given a cause in the form of Fortune, a *prosopopoeia* that reabsorbs accidents into a more purposive scheme by rendering them as effects of some superhuman agent.

Just as Egeon's narrative overdetermines the haps of his experience, the shorter descriptions of past events in the scenes that follow it suggest purpose where there is instead only an accidental convergence of circumstances. With the exception of the last scene, in which a final encompassing discourse is deferred until later, characters are often found describing the objectionable behavior of their perceived antagonists. The shift from surprise at confusing events to suspicion appears in the first exchange between Antipholus of Syracuse and Dromio of Ephesus at the end of the first act. When the Ephesian Dromio meets his master's brother, he is asked, "How chance thou art returned so soon?" The response has the disconnected character of a *parataxis* as clauses are reeled off without conjunction, a rhetorical license that assumes intimacy between the two characters:[21]

> Returned so soon? Rather approached too late.
> The capon burns, the pig falls from the spit.
> The clock hath struken twelve upon the bell;
> My mistress made it one upon my cheek. (1.2.43–46)

Like the clauses, the events described seem to follow in a quick sequence that could be either inevitable or arbitrary depending on one's point of view. While the story must be utter nonsense to Antipholus of Syracuse, it is absolutely clear to Dromio what connects these statements: dinner is burned and so is Adriana. Halfway through the speech Dromio begins to supply the logical connectors:

> She is so hot because the meat is cold.
> The meat is cold because you come not home.
> You come not home because you have no stomach.
> You have no stomach, having broke your fast;
> But we that know what 'tis to fast and pray,
> Are penitent for your default today. (1.2.47–52)

Dromio's first pass at an explanation parodies causal explanation, the initial *transumptio* giving way to a clever *gradatio* that figures the difficulty—perhaps even the irrelevance—of explaining the confusion with a chain of causes.[22] While his presentation tips spectators off to this important epistemological theme, it never puts in doubt the fact that individuals on stage are acting for reasons that they understand. Dromio has been beaten because Antipholus of Ephesus was late for dinner.[23] Adriana is wondering where her husband is, and Antipholus of Syracuse wants to know what happened to his money. Dromio wants something as well—to avoid another beating—and his presentation of the chain of causes, no matter how playful, shows that everyone involved is pursuing some purposive course of action.

Most of the language that follows this first contact in Ephesus reflects the problem of narrating past events that, although not immediately explicable, spontaneously suggest some hidden cause at work. When Dromio returns home from his beating in the market, for example, he receives another one after delivering this mannered rendition of past events:

> When I desired him to come home to dinner,
> He asked me for a thousand marks in gold.
> "'Tis dinnertime," quoth I. "My gold," quoth he.
> "Your meat doth burn," quoth I. "My gold," quoth he.
> "Will you come home?" quoth I. "My gold!" quoth he;
> "Where is the thousand marks I gave thee, villain?"
> "The pig," quoth I, "is burned." "My gold!" quoth he.
> "My mistress, sir—" quoth I. "Hang up thy mistress!
> "I know thy mistress not. Out on thy mistress!" (2.1.59–67)

Because Dromio cannot explain the events he has witnessed, his only way of rendering them is to repeat them somewhat mechanically. His speech is entertaining because it simply alternates between different perspectives without integrating them into a larger frame: the world seems a raw, unprincipled sequence of events in his description, an alienating bustle that only picks up speed when he tries to slow it down. That Dromio speaks of these events in such a mannered, self-conscious way suggests that he is familiar with this feeling: it is, in no small part, an expression of his status as a bondman. Knowing that he lacks the authority to impose an organization on events, Dromio perceives that any attempt to explain what has happened—which will involve boiling the sequence down into some causal nexus—is simply going to make matters worse. Instead, he tries to repeat what has happened blow by blow so that Adriana will understand that he is only reproducing the sequence of events rather than interpreting it. Thus, whereas Egeon's narrative in act one is a tissue of conjunctions, suggesting continuity and purpose, the speech by Dromio of Ephesus rattles along without them. There is a sense that Dromio must foreground the gaps in his story or risk being responsible for them (that is, it must appear to Adriana that the situation, not his incompetence, is the source of confusion). One gets the impression that the eclipsed connections—the causal "gaps" that everyone is ready to fill in this play—are a positive discontinuity sitting right on the surface of Dromio's recapitulation. This speech comes close to the "heart" of the mystery precisely because it avoids coming to terms with that mystery directly.

Few characters can resist the appeal of a deeper explanation, however. As the proverb reminds us, "every why hath a wherefore" (2.2.44), and in this play the catalogue of hidden causes is a long one, as I have indicated already. Witchcraft, adultery, jealousy, theft, madness, deception and headstrong disobedience are all entertained before errors made by accident come to explain the confusion. While several of the most immediate explanations are greeted as probable or improbable to various degrees, the possibility that the confusion is an effect of a unique set of circumstances and not deception or diabolical subversion seems beyond anyone's reach. Indeed, probable reasoning breaks down in Ephesus because the circumstances are so extraordinary, and the blindness of the characters to the accidents creating the confusion suggests that probable reasoning has found its rhetorical limit in this case.[24]

I say rhetorical limit because inevitably it is in speech that the probability of the different sources of the confusion is tested. Those tests are rarely conclusive, however, because no two people share enough of the same experience to allow any mutual recognition of that experience in the stories that are told about it.[25] The middle three acts are thus full of partial exchanges, interrogations, and accusations that preclude a sustained, narrative rendering of what has happened. While the story of the play is hurtling along, no one inside can get a story off the ground. Moreover, because speaking is an act, talking about the past in a certain way can itself become evidence that one is being deceptive or callous. The Dromios, for example, are regularly beaten both for what they have said in the past and for not holding their tongues when their masters remind them of what was said later on.[26] Talking about the past improbably is the insult that gets added to injury: it is assumed that the deceiver should have the decency to tell a good, believable lie if challenged. Thus Luciana counsels Antipholus of Syracuse to hide his infidelity in his speech, saying, "Be not thy tongue thy own shame's orator," (3.2.10) adding that "Ill deeds is doubled with an evil word" (3.2.20). The *enallage* of grammatical number here highlights the fact that stories about past actions are themselves actions, and yet they are rarely counted as such. To the extent that accidents in this play make for improbable matches between one person's memory of events and another's account of them, words come to multiply the past wrongs that they are expected both to confess and to assuage. There are thus not only accidental meetings of characters here, but accidental meetings of stories that keep the characters and the events they describe in some kind of sustainable disorder.

The stories that get told in act five are proper ones in the rhetorical sense. In their formal sophistication and reliance on legal convention, these narratives of deceit and trickery suggest that the proprieties and ornaments of rhetoric have come to stand in for—and so occlude—the absence of any deliberate wrongdoing in the past. The point becomes clear in the narrations of Adriana and Antipholus of Ephesus, both of whom describe the confusion to the Duke who will "determine" them. Adriana stops the Duke on his way to Egeon's execution, crying, "Justice, most sacred Duke, against the Abbess!" (5.1.134). The legal *narratio* that follows is meant, in good Ciceronian fashion, to describe the facts of the situation in a tight causal sequence.[27] What is entertaining about the story is its brevity: it is remarkably short considering the amount of confusion that must be explained. The broad summary sweep is sustained when independent processes are depicted simultaneously:

> Once did I get him bound, and sent him home,
> Whilst to take order for the wrongs I went,
> That here and there his fury had committed. (5.1.146–48)

The accommodation provided by the "whilst" both speeds the story along and allows the listener to think about the more hyperbolic "meanwhiles" of the story that have been witnessed on stage. "I went" at the end of line 147 intensifies this effect, representing a kind of temporal enjambment of one course of action (I went here and there to take order for the wrongs) with another (that his fury had committed). The speed of the narrative increases in her next sentence, which renders a particularly complicated set of reversals:

> Anon, I wot not by what strong escape,
> He broke from those that had the guard of him,
> And with his mad attendant and himself,
> Each one with ireful passion, with drawn swords,
> Met us again, and, madly bent on us,
> Chased us away; till, raising of more aid,
> We came again to bind them. (5.1.149–55)

Actions are described and, through repeated interjections, explanations given that condition subsequent actions. One can imagine Adriana breathlessly tacking on phrases like "Each one with ireful passion, with drawn swords," "madly bent on us" and "raising more aid," all of which provide the amusing sense that the complications of the story are testing the limits of her ability to press them into a spoken narrative.

The repeated hendiadys ("broke . . . and . . . met . . . and . . . chased us"), a trope that Adriana uses throughout the play, contributes further to the sense that the action is building in dizzying sequence (as well as foregrounding the rhetorical shorthand by which the "then" in narrative sequence is dropped). If Adriana were trying here to summarize what the audience itself has seen—accommodating all of the different circumstances that had to combine to create the situation she is now in—the narrative and rhetorical strain would probably be insurmountable.

When Antipholus of Ephesus arrives to demand justice, he bases his appeal on the Duke's past obligations:

> Justice, most gracious Duke, O grant me justice,
> Even for the service that long since I did thee,
> When I bestrid thee in the wars, and took
> Deep scars to save thy life; (5.1.191–94)

Here the Duke must remember or recognize himself in Antipholus's appeal to punish his wife, which he does when he tells Antipholus to "Discover how, and thou shalt find me just." The opening exchange establishes for all involved that this particular conversation will not be subject to the confusion that has attended other moments when Antipholus of Ephesus has tried to explain himself to an audience. The exchange also shows that Antipholus is engaged in a formal procedure of legal and rhetorical invention, since the Duke has asked the advocate to "discover" the cause of injustice in his speech. As with Adriana's careful exposition of events above, the formality of Antipholus's speech will be amusing precisely to the extent that it is superfluous—to the extent that it shows how the considerable resources of forensic rhetoric are, like the characters, completely at the mercy of circumstance.

In a procedure that the play's audience of law students would have recognized, Antipholus begins with a matter of fact, accusing Adriana of locking him out of his house. The Duke agrees that this is a "grievous fault" and asks Adriana if the charge is true. When she denies the charge and adduces a witness who swears that what she is saying is true, Angelo accuses both women of deceit ("They are both forsworn!" 213). With probable witnesses defending both sides of the contradiction, the trial is at an impasse. At just this moment, we get another studied *narratio*, this time from Antipholus of Ephesus, complete with apologetic *exordium* that meets the accusation that he is "mad" or "disturbed." Like Adriana's neat Ciceronian narration a few lines before, Antipholus's story consists of a pared down sequence of events all causally connected. As the Duke notes, Antipholus pleads "coldly," and the events that he describes seem to lead perfectly to his solution: he has been unfairly subjected to "shames and great indignities." The Duke recognizes that the facts at issue are now seriously in question ("Why, what an intricate impeach is this!" 270), but attributes the confusion to a mythological agent: "I think you all have drunk of Circe's cup," he says, and in so doing establishes that the right story has not yet been found to describe what is going on.[28]

The description by Antipholus of Ephesus of the "wrongs" done to him illustrates the entirely guileless way in which a narrative description translates an unexpected convergence of circumstances into a motivated series of events. Notably, it is around reported actions that the confusion peaks. When he and Balthasar meet the goldsmith, for example, Antipholus of Ephesus claims:

> There did this perjured goldsmith swear me down
> That I this day of him received the chain,
> Which, God he knows, I saw not. (5.1.227–29)

The audience too knows that the speaker never saw the chain, and in recognizing the truth in the goldsmith's report, they see it as a gap in the story rather than as evidence of deception. Yet there is no cunning manipulation of events or perspectives that strings events together in such a perfectly wrong way. The artistry—or some might say, the excess—of the plot creates a situation in which this narration could be an honest experience of events, could be wrong, and most important, could have occurred to the teller spontaneously. Circumstances, not purposive agents, have conspired in such a way that even the mere retelling of events accidentally supports the superfluous addition of causes and intentions as the "confederates" are identified and accused. This extraordinary situation tells us something fundamental about the linkage between linguistic ambiguity and rhetorical context in the production of comic laughter. A word like "Antipholus" or "Dromio," for example, may refer to several people, but it is the situation itself that must supply the wrong candidates for the right name. Laughter at such ambiguity is always also laughter at the facts of a particular situation: it is a sign that spectators have grasped the material and so the contingent link between words or stories and their possible contexts, which amounts to the recognition that any speech act in a social situation is subject to accidental or circumstantial forms of infelicity.[29] The philosophical upshot here is that it is not just the form and content of stories that are funny in a play like *The Comedy of Errors* but also the times and places in which those stories are delivered.

Like other narratives of past events, that of Antipholus of Ephesus is not completely wrong, but wrong enough that it will not clear up the confusion.[30] In supplying an end or "wherefore" for the actions taken against him, Antipholus of Ephesus indicates to those listening that error still prevails and that the play is not ready for its ending. One senses a straining within speech to bring about a conclusion in which narrative time, the time of speaking, and the time of the play converge. As the speech comes to a close, the bewildered Ephesian describes his escape from his abusers:

> Then all together
> They fell upon me, bound me, bore me thence,
> And in a dark and dankish vault at home
> There left me and my man, both bound together,
> Till, gnawing with my teeth my bonds in sunder,
> I gained my freedom, and immediately
> Ran hither to your grace, whom I beseech
> To give me ample satisfaction
> For these deep shames and great indignities. (5.1.246–54)

Like Adriana's story, her husband's contains staggered parenthetical remarks and concludes with a pivotal "Till" that brings it near the present moment of telling. As Antipholus shifts into present tense, however, it is clear that the ending described in his story—"ample satisfaction"—is not the comic satisfaction that will end the play itself.

That end does not come until about eighty lines later, when the twins meet face to face. On seeing the two side by side, the Duke exclaims:

> One of these men is *genius* to the other:
> And so of these, which is the natural man,
> And which the spirit? Who deciphers them? (5.1. 334–36)

The "and" that has been pushing the story forward now gains more significance, since characters realize that while they were discussing any one of the pairs, they were actually discussing one and the other. Emilia calls attention to the way in which speech can serve unexpected purposes, the way it accommodates both what one intends and what one does not:

> Speak, old Egeon, if thou beest the man
> That hadst a wife once called Emilia,
> That bore thee at a burden two fair sons.
> O, if thou beest the same Egeon, speak,
> And speak unto the same Emilia. (5.1.343–47)

When Egeon speaks to the Abbess, he will also be speaking to the woman described in her speech. The identities that can be remembered by these characters, memories that serve to individuate them when appearance cannot, are consolidated precisely when their stories can be shared. The coincidence here of memory, speech and speaking person thus marks an end to the immense disruptions that the twins and their accidental meetings have caused.

Upon hearing the Abbess plead to Egeon, the Duke dismisses the charges that have been made by declaring them the result of an "accident," suggesting the Ciceronian principle that crimes committed by chance may be admitted and then excused.[31] While this amounts to a final nod to the rhetorical tradition—a tradition that has arguably been present in every attempt to explain events on stage—the Duke's last speech also serves to remind audiences that a full accounting of events is forthcoming. On recognizing the circumstantial nature of the confusion, the Duke exclaims, "Why, here begins his morning story right" (5.1.348), and with this remark signals that he and those around him are ready to hear the story again—a story about accidents and the difficulty of recognizing them as such. What would such a story sound like? The Abbess provides the answer when, before the characters leave the stage to celebrate, she addresses the Duke:

> Renownèd Duke, vouchsafe to take the pains
> To go with us into the abbey here,
> And hear at large discoursèd all our fortunes,
> And all that are assembled in this place,
> That by this sympathizèd one day's error
> Have suffered wrong. Go, keep us company,
> And we shall make full satisfaction. (5.1.396–402)

The errors in this play are shared—"sympathizèd"—and in this turn of phrase we can see that the reservoir of suspicions and purposes that improbable events might be serving has been a communal one. When she points to "all those that are assembled in this place," the Abbess moves the story of the play into the room in which it is played. One can imagine the spectators at Gray's Inn recognizing themselves in her speech, picked out as they were in her round closing gestures. It was they, after all, who assembled with a pretend Prince and dignitaries to hear this entertaining tale. The final story, the end that has been deferred for so long, is thus the play that is being performed. And those who go to the Abbey to hear it from the beginning will, like its audience at the moment of performance, perhaps see the convergence of the past with the present as the play becomes a narrative of itself—of accidents as such—while the audience becomes that narrative's immanent destination. Happily, comically, the play seems to have hit upon a strategy for avoiding the ends and endings that accidents seem so readily to bring about. Understanding how that strategy works, however, requires that the tale be begun again.

Like the bodies that ricochet from one scene to the next, stories in *The Comedy of Errors* are always arriving at the wrong place at the right time. The ancient rhetorical principle of *kairos*, which holds that there is a perfect moment for persuasion, has been turned on its head in this play, in which the arrangement of onstage speakers and listeners seems almost mathematically calibrated to sustain the confusion.[32] While this quality of arrangement and contrivance might lead spectators to think about the hidden purposes of providence or the deity in the theater, the play's "analysis" of the situational and rhetorical sources of error suggests that this kind of deep providential reading is ultimately inappropriate. Like characters in the play, audiences are encouraged to see the mayhem on stage as harmless mischance rather than some portentous expression of divine control. They too must learn to avoid "ends," the play seems to be saying, recognizing the shaping power of circumstance in situations that seem to express some underlying purpose or order.

Such interpretive reticence is perhaps the natural response to farce, but it is also a consequence of seeing accidents repeatedly "disappear" in acts of narrative exposition. Indeed, when it depicts accidental causation as the indistinguishable twin of narrative causation, *The Comedy of Errors* engages some of the same philosophical issues surveyed in Chapters 1 and 2. Our examination of Aristotle and his Scholastic interpreters in those chapters suggested that narrative acquires a privileged status in the representation of accidents because it is indifferent to logical necessity and regularly ignores the causal links that we perceive in nature.[33] Narrative thus supplies a sense of continuity and progression that is not an intrinsic feature of the world being represented, but rather a "necessity" of the story as it is being told. As an extension of the learned tradition, *The Comedy of Errors* offers unexpected insights into this intimate relationship between narration and accidental causation. On the one hand, it suggests that narrative has an uncanny—and at times, hilarious—power to absorb whatever crosses its path into some meaningful whole. Farce thus picks up where Aristotelian metaphysics leaves off, since in staging and restaging accidental events for comic effect, it acknowledges the power of rhetoric and circumstance to shape "purposes" in situations that are not necessarily governed by some unitary cause. More figuratively, the play suggests that like the ocean or the woods, narrative context is the crossing point where purposes and expectations can meet in an entirely unregulated way. It is precisely because such crossings of story and context cannot always be governed by an intention or a rule that the act of narrating an accident is so fraught with difficulty in the play. This is not only true in the play, but *of* it, since the botched staging of *The Comedy of Errors* in 1594 and the subsequent trial of those "responsible" suggest that it was precisely this contingency of story on the situation in which it is delivered or performed that the play's early modern audience found intriguing.

In proposing that the play has philosophical content—which is to say, that its humor exploits and overturns metaphysical intuitions about the relationship between intention-bound speech and a rule-governed reality—I am not necessarily arguing that Shakespeare himself is a philosopher. Rather, I want to suggest that the early modern appreciation of the accident's rhetorical and metaphysical complexity was not limited to those who had made a detailed study of Scholastic distinctions and examples. Much of the subtlety of the Scholastic discussion is re-enacted and perhaps deepened in the farcical confusion that unfolds onstage in this play, in large part because farce requires the very situations and examples which put the philosophical problem of contingency in its most provocative (and most rhetorical) form. To what extent can accidental misunderstanding be avoided by careful description or probable reasoning? Shakespeare's audience of law students would have appreciated the thorny nature of such a question for professional reasons, and yet they may have left the performance with a measure of optimism. The extravagance of the farcical conceit makes the possibility of this kind of organized mayhem around accidents seem exceptional, the result of some bizarre pre-established harmony that is rarely found in the world. But to enjoy that extravagance, Shakespeare's audience had also to appreciate an underlying insight: that accident can never be completely banished from speech and the memories it delivers; like an interloping twin, it may always turn up in circumstances that cannot be foreseen. Due care or "cold" argument will not keep it in its place.

CHAPTER 4

'Hamlet' Interrupted

Toward the end of his famous soliloquy in act three, Hamlet's thoughts about life, death and the inhibiting powers of conscience are cut short. What shifts his attention—both Hamlet and the audience can see the cause plainly—is the appearance of Ophelia, now seen reading a devotional book in the place where Claudius and Polonius have instructed her to stand. The move from soul-searching to conversation takes place around a pause, the hero commanding himself to put private thoughts aside as he approaches Ophelia in prayer. Here is the passage:

> *Hamlet:* . . . Thus conscience does make cowards of us all;
> and thus the native hue of resolution
> Is sicklied o'er with the pale cast of thought,
> And enterprises of great pith and moment
> With this regard their currents turn away
> And lose the name of action.—Soft you now,
> The fair Ophelia.—Nymph, in thy orisons
> Be all my sins remembered.
> *Ophelia:* Good my lord,
> How does your honour for this many a day? (3.1.84–92)[1]

With the phrase "Soft you now," it is clear that Hamlet's attention has been caught from without. This shift in attention parallels the theme he has been developing in the soliloquy, that of enterprises abandoned. Hamlet's "regard" of Ophelia has interrupted his meditation, much as conscience and thought are described turning the currents of an enterprise awry.[2]

Hamlet is full of moments like this, when the action is discontinued and a character's attention is turned toward something new. Some of these interruptions are quite sudden, for example when the ghost disrupts the night watch in the first scene or when Hamlet leaps into the grave during Ophelia's funeral rites. We are apt to notice these shifts in a play like *Hamlet* because of their frequency and abruptness, but there is nothing exceptional about the redirection of a character's attention *per se* in Shakespeare's plays. Indeed, interruptions are only the most striking examples of a basic narrative strategy: the manipulation of a character's inner state of "regard" or attention toward or away from the events taking place on stage for dramatic purposes. We can think of this storytelling strategy as an inversion of what film does with the camera. Whereas classic Hollywood cinema can build tension in a story by pivoting point of view around the diegetic action, narrative tension in Shakespearean drama comes from the movement of "regard"—that inner angle or disposition of attention—with respect to the dramatic action. This strategy amounts to the theatrical management of attention, whereby players and playwright create meaning not just out of words or actions but also out of the degree of "regard" that characters give to events on stage.

"Regard" was itself a crucial category in Elizabethan writing and consciousness, since in turning the mind's eye toward this thing or that, one was assumed to value it or recognize its worth. As I will argue later, this equation of attention and feelings of moral obligation was particularly powerful in religious discourses at the turn of the seventeenth century, when the spiritual fact of belief or contrition was often associated with the act of "regarding" God's power and efficacy in the world. In late sixteenth-century England, a growing literature chronicled God's "judgement" on wayward sinners through unlikely "accidents," spiritual decay being described as a lack of proper "regard" for God's expectations and works—a deep sleep in which attention had ceased to resolve the image of divinity in the mind's eye. In saying that the theater manipulated and managed "regard" in this way, I want to suggest a historical link between the political and spiritual importance of attention and the particular vectors of its theatrical movement in Shakespeare's play.

Modern editorial practice often cues these inner movements of attention by adding stage directions (for example, "[Notices Ophelia]"), but Shakespeare seems to have assumed that the direction of attention could be gauged directly from the text through spoken formulae such as the exclamation. "Soft you now, the fair Ophelia," for example, tells spectators that Hamlet has stopped paying attention to his own thoughts and begun to regard something else. The actor on stage might look up from the floor and turn to face the woman—this too would be a reliable (but still conventional) marker. The meaning of Hamlet's words, as indicator of his thoughts, might also signal a shift, but thought should not be confused with attention. By talking about regard and its movement, I want specifically to distinguish the dramatic function of an exclamation like this one from its semantic value as a transcript of what Hamlet is "thinking." I am less interested here in what the exclamation says about the hero's thoughts than in the way the words mark a departure of regard from those thoughts to something else.

If we concentrate on regard and its movement in *Hamlet*, we see that it shifts in two fundamentally different ways. First, regard moves intradiegetically from one character or activity on stage toward another that has come to intervene. (Diegesis here refers to the collection of events enacted on stage.) When Polonius cries out during the closet scene, for example, it is clear who is doing the interrupting and where the attention should go. Regard also shifts extradiegetically, however, away from events taking place within the dramatic world toward an agency that has arranged those events for some kind of purpose. Unlike intradiegetic shifts in which attention moves toward an onstage prompter, these extradiegetic shifts originate within the individual, signaling his or her recognition that immediate circumstances are "in play," that they have been staged or arranged by an agency that indirectly controls them.

In *Hamlet*, this more radical form of interruption is associated with accidental events, outcomes that lack any apparent purposive cause in the agents which bring them about. Accidents are interruptions that do not necessarily refocus attention on an immediate interrupter; figuratively speaking, they are like skips on a record—sudden pops that make the listener aware of a world outside the music by calling attention to its source. *Hamlet* repeatedly stages this type of radical interruption, using the sudden movement of attention as a dramatic marker for changes taking place within the characters. The Prince's famous turn toward providence in act five for example, a crucial example of this process which I discuss at length below, happens when Hamlet begins to consider the unusual convergence of circumstances that enabled his return to Denmark. In its self-conscious use of accidental interruption as a dramatic device, *Hamlet* suggests a structural parallel between theatrical spectatorship and providential consciousness (with its attendant faculty of "conscience"), dependent as they both are on a knowledge that the world as a whole is contrived or artificial. This chapter explores that parallel and the shared form of knowledge or "conscience" it implies, moving outward from a discussion of accidental interruption in *Hamlet* to an examination of early modern religious literature which assumed that accidents could prompt a similar turn in regard, redirecting attention toward a divine source of meaning and obligation in the world.

In order to understand how such radical interruptions work, we will need to think of accidents not so much as attention shifters but attention reflectors, instances that catch individuals in the act of doing something which they must then recognize and acknowledge. I will try later on to provide a theory of how this kind of recognition works, arguing that in both theatrical and lived experience, regard shuttled in a constant state of "distraction" between the immediate causes of events and the all-encompassing purposes that those events might express.[3] As we will see, religious writers during the sixteenth century used accidents to interrupt this process of oscillation, forcing consciousness to catch itself dipping into an inarticulate belief in some purposive unity in the world. (Calvin thought that such a belief was universal, a seed of piety lodged in Christian and non-Christian souls alike.) A more controlled version of this process takes place in the theater, and if we look more closely at how "regard" moves in *Hamlet*, we can see how these worldly dynamics are imported into a theatrical space where they can be manipulated with an almost experimental precision.

While I plan to discuss a range of accidental events that occur in *Hamlet*, the most important for my argument about the movement of regard is Hamlet's rescue by pirates while he is traveling to England. Since at least the nineteenth century, this event has been treated as a kind of aesthetic rupture, or at least a highly artificial device that audiences must read in a willfully ironic mode. Coleridge found Hamlet's meeting with the pirates unique as a plot device because it resigned an "essential part of the plot" to mere accident.[4] A. C. Bradley too was aware of the unprecedented nature of the event, and in justifying the chance meeting at such a pivotal juncture he argues somewhat ingeniously that the accident is supposed to strike the reader as the reverse.[5] The utter improbability of the event, Bradley suggests, gives it an *obvious* sense of purpose—an ironic reversal that is then echoed in Hamlet's realization that the improbable circumstances of his rescue were manifestly arranged by God. Almost as soon as he has begun telling Horatio the story of his trip to England, Hamlet stops to think about the consequences of his own rashness:

> *Hamlet:* Sir, in my heart there was a kind of fighting
> That would not let me sleep. Methought I lay
> Worse than the mutines in the bilboes. Rashly—
> And praised be rashness for it; let us know
> Our indiscretion sometimes serves us well
> When our dear plots do pall; and that should teach us
> There's a divinity that shapes our ends,
> Rough-hew them how we will—
> *Horatio:* That is most certain.
> *Hamlet:* Up from my cabin . . . (5.2.4–13)

On the night that Hamlet retrieved the letters, the story suggests, it was his sleeplessness that gave him the opportunity to steal Claudius's letters away from his custodians. We do not hear what he did right away, however. With the digression that follows "rashly—," Hamlet leaves off the story of what happened during his journey to acknowledge the force that governed those events from above, a divinity that can "teach" of its presence and power precisely through those outcomes that exceed the human ability to determine them. With an almost breathless enthusiasm, the hero has turned his attention *away* from the events he is supposed to narrate toward a divinity that is shaping his ends. Horatio impatiently pulls the hero back on track when he agrees with the didactic conclusion, but it is clear from the animated way in which Hamlet is speaking that—like a man awake at midnight—his thoughts move readily to divine purposes.

This digression is one of the most dramatic moments in the play, suggesting for most critics that Hamlet has begun to come to terms with the limits of deliberate action or the overriding power of providence in human affairs.[6] While the significance of these lines is a perennial subject of debate, the sense that this is a moment of recognition seems beyond doubt. In reading this speech as a recognition that prefaces acceptance, critics are responding as much to what happens to attention in this scene as they are to what Hamlet is actually saying. Regard moves suddenly and extradiegetically with this digression, Hamlet's rescue narrative halting when he recognizes a divine purpose in the disposition of circumstances that allowed him both to alter Claudius's letters and to escape with pirates. Given the way in which the scene is staged, recognition and the shift in attention become one and the same gesture, so that the movement of regard and the meaning of its movement, supplied by Hamlet's invocation of providence, are united for the spectators in a startling yet believable way.

What we see in this moment of recognition is a theatrical version of the way in which individuals could be hailed or interpellated, to use Althusser's term, by providence in the world outside the theater.[7] While we may be accustomed to think of such hailings in a literal sense—a voice calling out, for example, saying "Tolle, lege"—a more subtle version of this recognition takes place when attention turns to God in response to coincidences or accidental occurrences. *Hamlet* models both kinds of call, in fact, since with the ghost we have an onstage voice that Hamlet must respond to with a mixture of filial and feudal obligation. The accident is a more subtle kind of appeal, however, because it requires Hamlet to turn his attention not to a person or thing but a diffused power that orders the circumstances around him.[8] With an accident, there is always a choice of where one can turn for an explanation; in turning to God, then, Hamlet appears spontaneously to recognize his role in the providential scheme.[9]

Hamlet's awakening stands in contrast to his past pronouncements, since earlier in the play he has acknowledged providence, but only as an afterthought or as some punishing order that he has no choice but to submit to. "The time is out of joint," he says in act one after taking his charge from the ghost, and then adds: "O cursèd spite, / that ever I was born to set it right!" (1.5.196–97). This rhetoric of providence as punishment is amplified after Hamlet kills Polonius, stabbing him blindly through the arras in Gertrude's chamber. Almost casually, by way of closing with his mother, Hamlet says that "heaven hath pleased it so, / To punish me with this, and this with me, / That I must be their scourge and minister" (3.4.162–64). Here providence is an indifferent calculus, a static balance of punisher with punishment expressed by the mirror symmetry of the figure of chiasmatic reversal. A detached form of pagan fatalism ("their scourge") also surfaces here, one that stands in opposition to Hamlet's obviously Christian recognition of God's providential care for the falling sparrow in act five. The divinity that "shapes" human "ends" in these early pronouncements is far from benign: instead of accommodating human ends, attending to the details of Hamlet's situation as it unfolds, providence legislates events before life even begins.

Until this exchange with Horatio, then, nothing that Hamlet has said about providence prepares spectators for this more intimate recognition that results from his accidental return to Denmark. The contrast is revealing not just as a measure of Hamlet's change of heart, which is the subject of most readings of this scene, but also as an illustration of the different kinds of providential consciousness that were possible during this period. While the pervasiveness of providential rhetoric (particularly around accidents) has suggested to many that a belief in providence was widespread during this period, that belief could be sincere or habitual, invoked in the spirit of consolation, with enthusiasm or with a certain resignation. We should not assume, I think, that the kind of providential consciousness on display in act five of *Hamlet* was adopted automatically during the period—as if such a consciousness were an idiom or figure of speech to be picked up in everyday usage. If the play gives us any indication of how this doctrine was embraced in the early modern period, there appears to have been a significant difference between those who could grudgingly affirm God's providential action and those who had given that belief some inner "stamp" of consent.[10] It is one thing to be told that God foresees and perhaps controls everything that happens (or even to fear that this must be the case); it is quite another to feel passionately, as Hamlet clearly does by the fifth act, that this doctrinal fact applies to you in particular.

Something must happen for providentialism to take hold, and accidents are the specific occasions on which early modern individuals recognize, in an intimate and personal way, their own participation in God's providential action. The most crucial aspect of that recognition is the shift in regard, one in which attention moves from events in this world toward the theatrical "ends" that are realized in them.

Providential Explanation of "Accidents" in Late Sixteenth-Century England

An irony that accompanies most providential interpretations of accidents during this period is that the more contrary such events are to expectation, the more necessary—from the standpoint of providence—they become. This connection between improbability and divinity was well established in Western Christianity when post-Reformation theologians in England began to formulate new ideas about providence during the late sixteenth century. Midway through the century, as we saw in Chapter 3, Jean Calvin had already begun to modify the conception of providence that he had inherited from Scholastic thinkers such as Thomas Aquinas and Albertus Magnus. These Catholic theologians, while struggling to understand what Aristotle called accidental events—encounters with pirates or robbers, unexpected meetings in the marketplace, fatal blows from falling objects—were less interested in what such events could teach the earthly spectator than in how accidents might be foreseen by God.[11] At issue was whether or not the lack of any regular cause for the accident made it impossible for God to know it would happen, a difficulty they resolved by saying that God knew the circumstances that determined accidental outcomes in the absence of the usual causes. The Scholastic God was thus a distant arranger of circumstances, and it was this aspect of his custody of the world that Calvin objected to.

For Calvin, as we have seen, God was more intimately present in the world and its events, his hand replacing Fortune's on the tiller of every earthly journey. God did not, as Calvin would say in the *Institutes*, launch people into the world like so many "tennis balls," reclining as he watched all of their paths collide in precisely the ways he had foreseen.[12] Rather, God was "vigilant, efficacious, operative, and engaged in continual action."[13] This "special providence" of God was at work even in accidents, but the "hidden counsels" that informed such events were not for human discovery. People could only wonder at accidents with a deepening sense of awe at God's inscrutable mastery of the world, understanding that "those things are subject to him which appear most fortuitous."[14] Significantly, Calvin suggests that the world is a providential theater in which apparently "chance" events strike the audience dumb, so powerfully do they evoke God's mysterious, governing power. For Calvin the difficulty was not so much that no one believed "accidental" or "fortuitous" events had a deeper purpose, but that they did not know what to do with that belief. Even pagans had a "carnal sense" that there was something more to accidents than mere chance. This response, he argues, is the native seed of providential belief which can be cultivated in all people with proper scriptural guidance.

During the late sixteenth and early seventeenth centuries, Scholastic and Calvinistic views were still exerting pressure on the interpretation of accidents. We can see aspects of these beliefs in England, where there were at least three kinds of providential interpretations that might have been applied to accidental events during this period. The first would be represented by Boethius, whose enormously popular *Consolation of Philosophy* was translated and reprinted several times beginning with George Colville's edition of 1556. As I pointed out in Chapter 2, this book contained all of the elements of the Scholastic position which was elaborated in the work of subsequent Catholic theologians. On this view, accidents were meetings of two or more causally independent chains of action, meetings that humans could know only as a matter of fact but that God nonetheless foresaw and arranged in advance by "disposing" circumstances in this or that way. A second, roughly Calvinistic view of providential custody was adopted by most Elizabethan English preachers.[15] On this view, what some ignorantly called "chance" or "fortunate" events testified to God's special and enduring care of the world, even though the specific link between those events and the divine purposes they served remained obscure and wondrous. Finally, a more robust interpretation is associated with religious writers such as Thomas Beard, William Ames and Phillip Stubbes, who did not believe that accidental events were this inscrutable; instead, accidents represented God's "judgements" on the specific moral choices of those whom they befell and could be studied as a kind of extra-biblical revelation.[16] It was these writers who took the theatrical analogy of providence to its limit, turning accidents into brutal illustrations of God's punishing and didactic control of events in the world.

What linked all of these views together was the notion that accidents were not really accidents to God, who either set them up in advance or presided over them the moment they occurred. To the extent that those talking about accidents in the late sixteenth century affirmed God's governance of such events, there was a great deal of continuity in their views. Elizabethan bishop Thomas Cooper thus makes an uncontroversial observation in a sermon published in 1580: "Whensoever misery or plague happeneth to man it cometh not by chance or fortune, or by a course of nature, as vain worldly men imagine, but by the assured providence of God."[17] The "vain worldly men" here could have been Epicureans, whose doctrine of the chance "swerve" of atoms and belief that the Gods do not care about human affairs were being revived with translations of Lucretius in the late sixteenth century. These views were anathema in Protestant religious circles, where accidents were more frequently thought to advertise God's interest in (and judgment on) human actions—a divergence from the more mystified posture that

Calvin recommended in these matters. From this new perspective, accidents were not simply test cases that faith or theological know-how needed to resolve; they were also signs to be heeded and, extending Calvin's metaphor, startling theatrical events that conformed to didactic purposes.[18] When Hamlet begins to talk about a "special providence" in act five, it is this specifically Protestant way of interpreting accidental events that both he and the play engage.

Keith Thomas, in describing how this brand of providentialism developed in the seventeenth century, points out that Puritan laymen were expected to keep records of the unexpected "mercies" or "deliverances" shown to them by providence. Any fortunate coincidence was noteworthy in this respect: "Hence the vogue for diaries and autobiographies chronicling the notable happenings in the writer's life—'accidents', as the astrologers called them."[19] Thomas quotes, in this connection, a treatise by R. Bolton, *Some generall directions for a comfortable walking with God,* in which the author finds that some people will conform to their holy duties when they fear they might be "seized upon with some remarkeable judgment, in their owne persons, families, or goods, by fire, robbery, tempest, ill successe, death, horrour, despaire, or other fearful accident."[20] The word "accident" here means "unexpected event" and, as we saw in Chapter 2, would have applied in this period to exactly the range of happenings described here. What is important about this trend is that it shows an increased awareness of some agency—calculating and potentially punishing—that is to be watched for in one's private life and meditated on conscientiously. Not only does God act for the edification of particular individuals, but the individual must pay attention to even the most trivial occurrences in hopes of discovering some edifying message.

Thomas Beard's popular *Theatre of Gods judgements* (1597), a translation of a French text by Jean de Chassanion, is a particularly significant document of the growing tendency to consult history and experience for signs of God's providential interest in the world.[21] In it Beard catalogues a variety of unpleasant ends that befall evil persons in both secular and ecclesiastical history; for example, a man who lapses into Catholicism during Mary's reign is poisoned by crow excrement that has been deposited on his head. Like others during the period, Beard decries those who do not observe the Sabbath. He gives the following two examples:

> Gregory Turonensis reporteth, that a husbandman who upon the Lords day went to plow his field; as he cleansed his plowshare with an iron, the iron stucke so fast into his hand, that for two yeeres he could not be delivered from it, but carried it about continually to his exceeding great paine and shame. Another profane fellow *without any regard of God or his service,* made no conscience to convey his corne out of the field on the Lords day in sermon time; but he was well rewarded for his godlesse covetuosnesse, for the same corne which with so much care he gathered togither, was consumed with fire from heaven [lightning], with the barne and all the grane that was in it. (195, italics mine)

By providing this kind of catalogue, Beard wants to show God's justice in the world, "to the end that the drousie consciences of Gods children might be awakened."[22] These unexpected accidents—neither of which would have been understood to be a miraculous suspension of any natural process—are understood as a divine response to an individual's lack of "regard" for God's will.

At least sixteen years earlier, Phillip Stubbes was already trying to point out how evildoers would be summoned to account for their misdeeds. In *Two wunderfull and rare examples of the undeferred and present approaching judgement . . .*, published in 1581, he describes how the servingman of a Master Pennell living in Lincolnshire "use to sweare, Gods precious blood . . . untyll at the last, it pleased God, to acite him, first with sickness, and last, with death." The calculated justice of the man's punishment is clear when blood, this time his own, streams from his fingers and nose.[23] What is interesting about Stubbes's commentary is that the punishment is meant to "acite," or summon, the man's attention in addition to causing him suffering. The effectiveness of this summons depends not just on his unexpected death, but also the coincidence of his manner of death with his habitual sin of swearing by God's blood.[24] The reader, presumably, will recognize the connection and so take heed of the example—seeing God's hand in the manner of punishment.[25]

While many of the books describing "Examples" of God's judgment simply alternate between particular sins and their eventual punishment, many of these accounts linger over ironic coincidences that make God's hand in the matter of his earthly judgments all the more striking. Samuel Saxey describes a "rare and lamentable Example" of God's judgment occurring in February of 1583, in which an adulterous couple are strangely burned one night in the house in which they have chosen to tryst. The same event appears to have been described in the 1583 edition of Phillip Stubbes's *Anatomie of abuses,* in which Spudeus and Philoponus discuss a usurer named Ratsurb who is struck down by God during an adulterous assignation with a woman. The man's arm is burned almost completely off, while the woman's abdomen and, presumably, her womb are consumed by the fire.[26] The fire could have burned anything, of course, but in this case it seems to have sought out the particular guilty limbs and organs. One becomes aware of the odd, implicating logic involved in this mode of explanation in merely citing such examples. How, for example, does someone recognize the correspondences between usury or adultery and the circumstances of this couple's death without already in some sense believing that those practices are sinful? There is something coercive about even recognizing that an accident accomplishes an end in an instance like this, since in doing so one seems to give assent to the underlying moral assumptions which make that outcome noteworthy in the first place.

Another example of divine judgment through accident was the sudden fall of a scaffolding that killed seven people who were watching a bear baiting one Sunday in Paris Garden, London, in 1583. Their guilt seems more obvious because they were caught in the act—interrupted, as it were, in the midst of their debauchery. In the report of the accident made by John Field, readers are exhorted to pay attention to the judgment of God as it appears in this and other misfortunes:

> O *England* repent, thou that hast tasted of so many blessings, and yet hast provoked God with so many sinnes. O *London* repent, thou that hast sit as a Lady & Queene over thy neighbor Cities, to whom the Lord hath given beside temporal blessings these precious jewels: sending thee many messengers to warne thee, to preach unto thee, and to comfort thee: *but thou has not regarded the day of thy visitation*.[27] (last italics mine)

Throughout this scathing treatise, Field criticizes the blindness of Londoners to God's dissatisfaction with Sabbath breakers, finding greatest fault with those "that have made no regarde of these things."[28]

Field's use of the word "regard" here is of a piece with a more pervasive rhetorical strategy in sixteenth-century "judgement" literature to equate belief in God's providence with attention to divine purposes in unusual events of all kinds. Turning one's attention toward something has a range of meanings in this period: "regard" confers value on the thing regarded, signals interest, awareness, deference and even obligation—a range that made it attractive to reformers.[29] In 1570, for example, this passage from a letter from Jean Calvin prefaces an account of an Italian man named Francis who was struck down with madness immediately after renouncing his reformed beliefs:

> How frowarde our mynde is in judgynge thee workes of god, & how croked a judgemente we have, it doth ryght well appeare by thys, that whereas he sheweth so many examples one after an other in punishing the wickednes of man, *yet many do sleightly passe over, or regarde the same*, yea, some playnely scorne them, other suppose them to come by chaunce: and finally, all men sodainly forget them.[30] (italics mine)

Clearly the ascription of such events to chance is a spiritual error for Calvin, since in doing so the spectator ceases to pay any attention whatsoever to the purposeful nature of such prodigious events. What these accounts of unusual judgments must do instead is to foreground divine purpose by narrating observed calamities or preservations in a way that links them, circumstantially, to some prior sinful or virtuous act.

Of abiding concern in these case studies of affliction, particularly in their prefaces, was the need to see God's providential action in what was somewhat unthinkingly—and certainly less piously—referred to as "misfortune." In a study of Job published by Henry Holland in 1596, for example, the author writes in a chapter on the "Use of the doctrine of Gods providence":

> We learne here to be patient in afflictions, considering the hande of our God is present with us, and his eyes are ever upon us: let our eyes, the eye of our faith, be fixed and fastened upon him, and quietly let us say with Job, As it pleaseth the Lord, so it came to passe, blessed bee the name of the Lord.[31]

Holland's phrase—"the eye of our faith"—makes clear the metaphorical connection that was being made between literal seeing and the kind of spiritual attentiveness that these writers were trying to cultivate. Yet in arresting the eye of faith, these writers were not only hoping to produce spiritual awaking. Such attentiveness was also a form of governance, as we learn from the Preface to Beard's translation of Chassanion's *Theatre of Gods judgements*. Here the author justifies the cataloguing of misfortunes that befall reprobates because such a catalogue can "set before our eyes" the threatened punishment for sinning:

> And so for this cause also God himselfe our soveraigne and perfect lawgiver, that hee might fashion and fit us to the mould of true and solid vertue, useth oftener negative prohibitions than affirmative commandements in his law: to

the end above all things to *distract and turne us from evill,* whereunto we are of our selves too much inclined. And as by this meane sinne is discovered and made known unto us, *so is the punishment also of sinne set before our eyes* by those threatnings and curses which are there denounced: to the end, that whome the promises of life and salvation could not allure and persuade to do well, them the feare of punishment (which followeth sinne as a shadow doth the body) might bridle and restraine from giving them over to impietie. (A4r–v, italics mine)

Beard's rhetorical equation of sight with obedience here suggests the regulatory role that such a watchfulness can play in bridling sinful behavior when those same punishments are observed in the world. William Perkins, writing about God's providential care of the world in his *A golden chaine,* published in 1600, explains this link between observing God's providence and self-restraint:

If men were perswaded that the Prince had an eye every where, doubtlesse many subjects in England would walke more obediently to the lawes of the land then they doe: and durst in no wise work such villianies as are daily practised. Well, howsoever it is with earthly princes, yet this all-seeing-presence is least wanting in God: he hath an eye every where: wheresoever thou art, there God beholdeth thee.[32]

Perkins elaborates an important consequence of the doctrine of providence here in this chapter devoted to the topic: in recognizing God's activity in the world, an individual would at the same time become subject to a perpetual and regulating scrutiny of his or her every action.[33]

While many of the "lamentable" or "marvelous accidents" described in the "judgement" literature were singled out because they occurred only rarely, what was spiritually arresting about a judgment was the element of irony or purpose that could be seen informing events that might otherwise be only circumstantially related. Clearly heaviness could bring down a scaffolding, plague could kill, and earthquakes, floods or lightning could destroy the cities they struck. What needed to be explained in these events was not so much their immediate causes but the fact that they happened to this particular person or place instead of some other. While Aristotle would have simply resigned such connections to the philosophical dead end of chance or accident, a distinctly Christian brand of poetic justice was being urged on the world toward the end of the sixteenth century. Being out on a Sunday to watch some questionable entertainment on precisely the same day when the scaffolding fell, for example, would have shown—because such an event could have just as easily happened a day later—that it was God who decided that the scaffolding should fall on this day rather than another. These accidents appeared to be a divine interruption of sinful activity—a "judgement," "rod," or "scourge" depending on the circumstances.[34] Such interruptions did not necessarily need to be contrary to the causes at work in nature; if they were, they would have been called miracles. Rather, the kind of "judgements" that were interesting religious writers in this period were aimed directly at the consciences of those whose regard has ceased to focus on God's expectations and so needed to be redirected. A sea did not need to be parted and the sun did not need to stop in the sky to accomplish this. Striking or ironic coincidences would be enough to summon the wayward back to the fold.

Shifting Regard

I have focused extensively on this religious literature to show how a particular tautological circle—where the hidden purpose of accidents entailed a belief in providence and vice versa—could be closed when an individual turned his or her attention to the divine purposes that accidents might serve. In England during the late sixteenth century, there was enormous competition for attention where accidents were concerned, since in regarding God in the accidents of the world, one might be understood to recognize one's moral obligations to a divinity who was actively evaluating the behavior of individuals.[35] As the boom in "judgement" literature suggests, earthly authorities were eager to highlight the most conspicuous examples of God's providential activity for those who had not yet recognized it. Ideally, however, the impetus for such a turn would be found somewhere in the individual. Hamlet's famous "divinity" speech in act five is powerful precisely because it shows him making the connection between his own rashness and God's preparedness for himself. The digression within the story he is telling serves as audible evidence that he has paused to recognize something, that he has responded to some sign of God's presence in the world that only a believer would know how to read.

When we bring the emerging discourse of accidental judgments to bear on this moment in the play, we can imagine how striking the transition from a more doctrinal acquaintance with God's providence to passionate belief would have been to the spectators who watched it taking place. Such a move would have both dramatic and theological value:

the turn to "regard" providence would have all the hallmarks of a spontaneous recognition—something that is exploited for dramatic purposes in this scene—but also, and more important, would confirm that an inner sense of obligation was subjecting the individual to a governing, divine power.[36] This moment becomes even more interesting when we see how *Hamlet* puts the spectator in a position to make a parallel turn. When the spectator learns of Hamlet's rescue by pirates, he or she may suddenly begin to consider the "extradiegetic," authorial purposes that such an "accident" might be serving. By pivoting Hamlet's turn toward God on the same event that points the audience toward the playwright, *Hamlet* introduces a comparison between the providential guidance being asserted within the dramatic world and the authorial control which is presumed to govern it from without.

Such a comparison can only be supported by an event that audiences recognize as indirectly contrived, one that shifts attention away from the immediate action and toward a "providential" agent directing the action in the theater. While the pirate rescue does not constitute a novel appearance of the author's hand in the play—the ghost, after all, would have struck audiences as equally contrived given the well-worn conventions of Elizabethan revenge tragedy—the episode is nevertheless an obvious token of the author's designing activity and the indirect means by which his purposes are accomplished. One hallmark of authorial contrivance in this episode is the fact that spectators do not see the pirate rescue take place, but instead hear it narrated in a letter. Both of these means of relating the event, the narration and the letter, are expedient theatrical devices that playwrights regularly use to bring extraneous knowledge to characters and the audience.[37] News of the encounter, moreover, seems almost smuggled in from outside of the world of the play, as if a generic field stops at the west coast of Denmark and the sea surrounding it is governed by the quick-bending laws of romance, pirates swooping in just in time to take the hero somewhere else. The pirates literally come from elsewhere, from the sea, from the romance, even—when we consider Shakespeare's audience of the early 1600s—from contemporary political and commercial concerns about the effects of piracy on the shipping trade.[38] All of these factors converge on the accident at sea to invest it with a purpose in excess of the one it immediately expresses: the aim of the pirates to obtain some favor from the king.

We could say that the pirate rescue "points" toward the author, but a more accurate description is that the improbable accident *interrupts* a relatively smooth oscillation between a spectator's consciousness of events autonomously evolving on stage and, what is only a potential contradiction, an awareness that these events have an artificial unity imposed by the author. When the pirate rescue brings these opposed forms of consciousness together, the oscillation stops and spectators are "caught" playing a double game—evaluating events as an independent fact of the world and as a "device" that has been imposed on that world for a reason. This juggling process, which is a possibility condition of the accident's interpellating power, is completely overlooked when spectatorship is described in terms of "belief" in a theatrical "fiction," since the term "belief" suggests that one is either totally won over by a dramatic world or left to stand outside of it in skeptical denial. Like other plays in the Shakespearean canon, *Hamlet* is aimed at a spectator who stands on both sides of the fiction, a spectator for whom consciousness in the theater is a state of controlled distraction.

When we examine the judgment literature that surrounds the play, we see that individuals hailed by providential accidents in the world are being actively urged into a similar state of "distraction"—not one of madness, but of divided attention. The Puritan theologian William Perkins makes this point in an astonishingly literal way when, in a treatise on providence, he implores individuals to look on the world with one eye and to God with another:

> wherefore as we looke on the thing done, so we must also in it, labour to see and acknowledge the good pleasure & appointment of God. As for example: a mans house is set on fire, and all his goods consumed; this very sight would make him at his wits end: but now as he beholds this event with one eie, so with the other eie he must at that very instant looke upon Gods blessed providence.[39]

Turning one eye toward God in the "very instant" of disaster is, according to Perkins, a way for the individual to "acknowledge" something which he or she already knows but is too lazy (or perhaps shocked) to look for. Like other theologians during this period, Perkins understands that the greatest difficulty he has in advancing the case for providence is that of making individuals aware of their capacity for divided attention, to remind them that on some level they are already aware of a force in the world that has the power to invest accidents with some overriding purpose.

Perkins uses a familiar term to describe this providential consciousness and the knowledge it possesses: "God knowes perfectly all the doings of man, though they be never so hid and concealed: and man by a gift given him of God, knowes togither with God, the same things of himselfe: and this gift is named Conscience."[40] When we understand conscience in this way—as a spectator within the spectator, one who possesses a special knowledge shared by God—we realize how closely providential consciousness resembles the mobile consciousness of the theatrical spectator. The two are united in their possession of a similar knowledge: both know that the world as a whole is contrived, no matter how autonomous it may seem, and both can exercise that knowledge in the interpretation of events which must be viewed "distractedly," from at least two perspectives simultaneously. This quasi-divine knowledge possessed by the early modern providential spectator of accidents stands in stark opposition to the mere circumstantial knowledge that the Scholastic theologians attributed to those who saw them take place.

In *Hamlet*, this capacity for "distraction" is exercised again and again in scenes that depict attention moving away from the immediate action and latching on to some hidden agency or purpose which is directing the action. By examining several of these scenes in succession, I want now to deepen the analogy offered above and suggest that we understand early modern providential consciousness as a more portable variety of the kind of "distraction" that held sway in the theater. While this analogy is implicit in both the play and the providential literature that surrounds it, the parallel between the providential and theatrical spectator is best grasped through a precise set of terms and examples—those terms and examples which the play offers as it stages accidental interruptions in a variety of theatrical frames. I will be reading the play, then, as both an extended performance of the extraordinary mobility of theatrical consciousness and, later on, a theatrical experiment that tests the limits of spectatorial knowledge as audiences attend to events unfolding in the play.

One of the most striking instances of theatrical awakening occurs soon after the encounter I discussed in the opening of this chapter, when Hamlet discovers Ophelia in prayer. Before the meeting takes place, Polonius sets his daughter in her place and gives her instructions on how to act, arranging the scene much as a director might block the action for the stage. She is to read a prayer book alone, which will make it seem as though she is not looking for Hamlet when the two meet. Claudius describes Polonius's stratagem as a staged accident, one that will test his suspicions about the sources of Hamlet's unusual behavior. Asking Gertrude to leave the scene, he explains the plan.

> Sweet Gertrude, leave us too;
> For we have closely sent for Hamlet hither,
> That he, as 'twere by accident, may here
> Affront Ophelia.
> Her father and myself, lawful espials,
> Will so bestow ourselves that, seeing unseen,
> We may of their encounter frankly judge,
> And gather by him, as he is behaved,
> If't be th'affliction of his love or no
> That thus he suffers for. (3.1.29–38)

We can think of this event as the theatrical precursor of a Baconian experiment described in the next chapter: an attempt to access hidden truths by staging an "accident" and then observing what happens. By the end of the interview, Claudius is convinced that Hamlet's troubles do not spring from love, and so it appears that the experiment has been a success. This is not entirely the case, however, since the subject of the experiment seems to learn something about the experimenter as well.

In the midst of his tirade against the breeding of sinners, Hamlet suddenly shifts focus and asks, "Where's your father?" (3.1.131). This of course is precisely the question to ask, since Polonius, while "unseen," is nevertheless present to observe the encounter with his daughter. More important, Polonius is present in Hamlet's consciousness, a new object of attention surfacing in the midst of an argument about honesty's commerce with beauty. As with Hamlet's earlier encounter with Rosencrantz and Guildenstern, when he immediately grasps the king's role in bringing his friends to Denmark to sound him out, Hamlet is quite ready to suspect the staged or contrived nature of this "accidental" encounter with Ophelia. There is no way to be certain from the source texts whether or not he actually knows that Polonius is watching, but the spontaneous movement of regard in this scene—the way it gravitates toward the agent who is staging this "accident" for a deliberate purpose—charts the trajectory for the more decisive flight it will make in act five.[41]

Perhaps the most dramatic moment of awakening takes place during another "test" of sorts: the performance of *The Mousetrap*. The scene is arranged so that the audience of *Hamlet* can observe both a target spectator (Claudius) and his surroundings, taking in the dual scene unfolding on the stage and in the stands. When he is devising this scene, Hamlet remarks that occasionally spectators at a play will "by the very cunning of the scene" be "struck so to the soul" that they proclaim their guilt (2.2.579–80). The word "cunning" here is rich with associations of deviousness, craft, and skillful contriving during this period, but also has the meaning of "knowing."[42] The semantic range of this term suggests that it is not just skillful representation of action that will strike Claudius's guilty soul, but—figuratively—a knowledge which that representation expresses. This semantic resonance is picked up again at the end of Hamlet's speech, where the hero says, "The play's the thing / Wherein I'll catch the conscience of the King" (2.2.593–94). Here too the term "conscience," with its early modern meaning of knowledge and awareness, serves as a gloss on the nature of the theatrical trap that is being prepared for Claudius: the play is literally going to capture the King's attention as he watches, grappling deviously with what he knows but is unwilling to reveal.

The idea that artistic "cunning" and "conscience" might be connected, suggested by their mutual association with knowledge, can be further elaborated as a metaphor for the shared status of authorial and spectatorial consciousness in the theater. Building on the semantic logic of Hamlet's imagery, we might say that the theatrical fiction of Hamlet's description becomes the common mental space of its author and audience, somewhat as Newton's mechanical universe, in a very different context, becomes the sensorium of God. In that common place—"wherein" events unfold and actions are taken—the author's knowledge of how to "invent" or "contrive" overlaps with an audience's ability to invest those happenings with significance. The language of devising, "cunning" and "conscience" throughout the play could thus be read as gesturing toward a profound fantasy of intersubjectivity within the theater, one in which authorial knowledge of how to create a fiction perfectly coincides with an audience's knowledge of how to interpret it.

When this fantasy is brought to bear on the scene in which *The Mousetrap* is performed for the Danish court, we discover that Hamlet is himself pushing toward some mediated form of shared consciousness with his antagonist. Given the way the performance is set up, Hamlet is not really a spectator of the play but a student of Claudius's guilt, his eyes riveted on the King's face as the "circumstance" of his father's death (as reported by the ghost) is enacted on stage. Shakespeare has placed the audience of *Hamlet* in a similar position: it must test a character's internal state (here guilt) by the evidence of his attention, an evaluation that is a staple of theatrical interpretation but that has been raised, in this scene, to the level of a dramatic crux. Neither audience is disappointed, for when Claudius proves unable to watch the performance, interrupting the scene in which Player Lucianus pours poison into the Player King's ear, both sets of onlookers witness an extraordinary recognition. Claudius the spectator has, in taking his eyes off the performance, bracketed the action on stage in its totality and identified it as a model or digest of what he has done in the past. He has ceased, in other words, to follow the story and instead focused his "regard" on Hamlet, who at that very moment is glossing the scene and announcing what will come next. Given the way Shakespeare has set up this scene, the play becomes a message, an intimate communication between undeclared opponents, strangely public but also completely private. It is as if, with everyone watching, the Prince has leaned over and whispered to the King: "I know what you've done."

The *Mousetrap* scene illustrates the dynamics of distracted spectatorship in an extraordinarily precise way, since it allows the audience to stand outside the frame of the play-within-the-play and observe the circulation of "regard" around the entire scene. Once again an accident is associated with the moment of interruption, not as an event onstage, but as a possible explanation for the likeness of events in *The Mousetrap* to crimes that Claudius has committed. We can think of the convergence of onstage fiction and personal memory as if it were itself an event, like the discovery of treasure while digging a well or the arrival of twins in the same place.[43] This resemblance is not dismissed as a coincidence or mere chance, however. Instead, the similarity of fact and fiction engages another consciousness within the King, a memory of the depicted crimes and a sense of the larger situation in which he finds himself. The immediate presence of others around him is a powerful fact of Claudius's consciousness in this scene, one that we should not slight by reading the scene in strictly moral terms. While the king may be absorbed in the drama, he is also surrounded by courtiers, friends and—foremost among his concerns—an enemy whose melancholy presents a "danger" to himself and the state (3.1.168).

There is always something of this crowd present in the mind of the spectator, and I would argue that the *Mousetrap* scene is only one of many illustrations in *Hamlet* of a basic fact of theatrical consciousness: it is subject to competing claims for attention and responds to pressures that are not immediately present in the "illusion" presented on stage.[44] Providentialists were crucially concerned with this other half of theatrical consciousness and worked to enhance it, recognizing as they did that the individual's capacity for controlled distraction was precisely what allowed a theatrical knowledge of God's design to exercise its regulatory role on interpretation and, ultimately, individual behavior. Theatrical "conscience" is concerned with more than right and wrong, however, and as we chart the vectors of theatrical consciousness in this scene, we should not ignore the fact that personal memory (Claudius's knowledge of his fratricide) and political history (the explosive secret of his usurpation) are shown to be equally powerful sources of diversion, equally capable of commanding the King's attention and concern. When we set Claudius's political concerns alongside his guilt, this scene becomes an allegory for the mobility of early modern theatrical consciousness in general, a consciousness that was quite capable of circulating outside the boundaries of the theatrical "illusion" to engage an array of religious, political and cultural concerns.[45]

The scene with Claudius also extends the parallel I have been making between theatrical consciousness and religious conscience, suggesting that they both depend on a common capacity for interruption. We see that capacity displayed for the last time when Laertes reveals the secret of Claudius's guilt after the rapier contest has ended. The entire scene has been contrived by the King as a kind of secret (but nonetheless public) execution of his nephew, an exercise in political and theatrical "providence" that conceals the nature of the revenge being taken on Hamlet by making his death appear a mishap.[46] Before the contest takes place, the audience watches Claudius cast about for a plan that will allow Laertes to kill his father's murderer. The process of invention unfolds spontaneously as the King—now perhaps a symbolic surrogate for Shakespeare as he plots the ending of the play—considers the new information contained in Hamlet's letter:

> If he be now returned,
> As checking at his voyage, and that he means
> No more to undertake it, I will work him
> To an exploit, now ripe in my device,
> Under which he shall not choose but fall;

> And for his death no wind of blame shall breathe;
> But even his mother shall uncharge the practice
> And call it accident. (4.7.62–69)

By using the word "device," Claudius alerts us to the fact that it is a particular faculty that is responsible for imposing purposes on a set of circumstances which are "ripe" for arrangement.[47] This faculty is similar to the one that interprets accidents as the expression of some will: both see a potential purpose in the disposition of agents in the world, but in the case of "device," that purpose is shaped into a plan for action.

The rest of the interview focuses on the details of the plan, Claudius taking extra precautions to create a backup plot (that of the poisoned drink) which will kill Hamlet if the first plan happens to "blast in proof"[48] (4.7.130). In attempting to pre-empt accidents, however, Claudius ends up ensuring that they will happen: the cup filled with poison never makes it to Hamlet's lips, but is instead taken up by Gertrude, who toasts her son's fortunes after he has scored a hit.[49] Another accident occurs when Hamlet gets the rapier from Laertes and stabs him with it in the skirmish.[50] Once these mishaps have occurred, Claudius's "providence" appears to have reached its limit: he cannot control the trajectory of the plot once it has been launched, nor can he physically intervene to stop Gertrude from becoming one of its casualties.

As one mishap follows another, spectators are able to compare the reactions of the two "contrivers" as they respond to the unfolding disaster. In staging this comparison, the play offers a dramatic contrast between two characters, one of whom still has the capacity to interpret accidents as part of some larger organizing scheme, and another who is dull to their significance. Claudius, for his part, is completely unavailable for any kind of ironic reflection on the accidental turn of events in this scene. Even after he has been mortally stabbed with the poisoned foil, he does not pause to recognize that his treacherous gambit has failed. "O, yet defend me, friends, I am but hurt" (5.2.277), he says to the courtiers, and in so doing displays a "conscience" completely fortified against the irony of this reversal.[51] Laertes, however, is stunned into confession and self-judgment by the failure of the plot. When Osric turns to him for an explanation of what is happening, Laertes tells him: "Why, as a woodcock to mine own springe, Osric. / I am justly killed with mine own treachery" (5.2.260–61). This formula is then repeated later, in his dying words, when Laertes says of Claudius, "He is justly served; / It is a poison tempered by himself" (5.2.280–81). Both of Laertes's declarations, articulating as they do the dramatic irony of this moment, signal for the audience that conscience has become fully engaged.[52]

This will be the most explicit judgment passed on events taking place at the end of the play, since Horatio offers only a preface to the longer tale of "accidental judgments, casual slaughters," a preface which specifically avoids the suggestion that those mishaps are redeemed by any overriding principle of justice. Hamlet too is mute on the question of the significance of what has happened, having left his providential reflections behind for concerns with his legacy and the election of a future king.[53] Someone must, Hamlet reminds the audience, explain what has happened to those who have no knowledge—and so historically, no memory—of Claudius's crimes:

> You that look pale and tremble at this chance,
> That are but mutes or audience to this act,
> Had I but time—as this fell sergeant Death
> Is strict in his arrest—O, I could tell you—
> But let it be. Horatio, I am dead;
> Thou liv'st; report me and my case aright
> To the unsatisfied. (5.2.287–93)

Once again, Hamlet and *Hamlet* are about to be interrupted, death bringing the story to a precipitate close. The Prince's last sentence will actually trail off unfinished, halted by a final declaration: "—the rest is silence" (5.2.311).

It is significant that the final moments of the play are addressed to a spectator, one who presumably pales and trembles at the "chance" that has left so many of the major characters dead. When Hamlet gestures toward the "you" who "looks" in this scene, the play is working in the most traditional of ways to solicit the fear and pity of an audience who must now consider (in good Aristotelian fashion) the accidental outcome's tragic meaning. As the indirect addressee of this final invitation, the audience of *Hamlet* the play is hailed by the same silent imperatives that have turned the regard of characters throughout. Accidents are once again a subtle appeal to read for irony, an invitation to transpose the purposelessness of mere coincidence into a poetic register where its hidden meaning can be grasped in a kind of deferential awe, precisely the kind of awe that Calvin recommended in such situations. Accidents are also, from our critical perspective, an invitation to become a subject of the knowledge that one is in the theater, a knowledge that is the structural condition for the recognition of deeper purposes in tragic misfortune.

This form of subjection was probably not, as the term might suggest, a form of inhibition. Indeed, becoming the subject of a distinctly theatrical brand of providence was one of the pleasures that early modern audiences went to the theater to experience. Such an experience, premised as it was on a submission to the diffuse will of another, could become pleasurable as soon as it was voluntary: it followed upon payment of the price of admission. The invitation to wonder at tragic accidents at the end of *Hamlet* raises important questions, however, about the relationship between the implied spectator of this play and the subject of providential ideology as I have been theorizing them here. If, as the play suggests, theatrical and providential consciousness are structurally identical, does it then follow that a spectator who responds to the tragic crescendo at the end of *Hamlet* is exercising, and so perhaps deepening, his or her capacity for providential "interruption" outside of the theater?

On some level, yes. It is hard to imagine an early modern spectator refusing the invitation to wonder providentially at accidents at the end of *Hamlet*, particularly when the considerable forces of tragic theater and Reformation theology were so perfectly arrayed to compel such a response. Faced with such an ending, an audience steeped in the religious culture of Calvin, Beard and Perkins would have experienced a profound convergence of its habitual modes of attending, finding in the providential theater of this play an almost exact image of its own tendencies to probe accidents for their providential meaning. Even an audience member who sympathizes with Horatio's long-suffering, Stoic attitude at the end of the play must nevertheless adopt the habits of attending that characterize the providential spectator of this period. In its repeated alignment of divine and dramatic "contriving," moreover, *Hamlet* deepens the theatrical model of divine providence that so powerfully transformed the early modern capacity for tragic awe into what Calvin regularly referred to as a "fear" of God. By deepening the link between this model and the stage, the play cannot help but affirm the hierarchical model of Elizabethan society in which divine providence spills over into the fountains of royal governance and finally into the cups of God's subjects. The conclusion of *Hamlet,* no matter how complex in its irony and layerings, provides a lasting pathos for that hierarchical vision, particularly when the usurper Claudius is finally forced off the throne by an "accident" that can itself be read in providential terms.

And yet, the providential order that unfolds in *Hamlet* unfolds in a specific place, the theater, and so like the theatrical performance itself must on some level be experienced as provisional.[54] While I doubt that the play had the effect of "unmasking" Christian providence as something unreal or illusory, its self-conscious depiction of accidents would have temporarily bracketed these events as a phenomenon of the theater and so an expression of its particular powers.[55] In *Hamlet,* those powers are not limited to the capacity for ordering events from afar—as if the theater is simply an instrument for action—but extend to its capacity for testing, trial and discovery through the manipulation of circumstances.[56] There is no reason why some of Shakespeare's spectators may not have grasped the play as itself a trial of this sort, one that tested their own knowledge of the theater, its conventions and its reigning provisional deity.

How would such a trial or experiment work? When *Hamlet* deliberately reshuffles the stock tropes of tragedy—not simply the trope of the fateful accident, but also the ghost, the play within the play, the woman mad with grief—it asks spectators to recognize these elements as a version of other moments in the theater. As one of many such tokens that make reference to other imaginary experiences (rather than experiences in the world), accidents serve as an "indirection" or experiment with theatrical consciousness, a gambit in a game of intelligence between a playwright and spectator in which each must guess at what the other knows about events on stage. To the extent that such a knowledge of other performances must be solicited rather than supplied by the playwright, the balance of providential power temporarily shifts away from some (highly orthodox) center of authorial control toward a spectator who must complete the "illusion" by recognizing its deferred origin in other instances of performance.[57] As the balance tips in this direction, *Hamlet* becomes less an illustration of the theatrical nature of providence and more of an experiment with the radically commutative nature of experience in the theater—an attempt to understand how that experience carries over from one performance to the next and in doing so creates a contingent play across them. An individual so hailed by devices like the accident and ghost thus becomes a citizen of the theater rather than a subject of God.

There are reasons why spectators might have found this experimental conception of theatrical contriving more appealing than the providential one, since the providential reading of the play, no matter how reassuring, would nevertheless have generated a certain amount of anxiety in the Christian spectator. Problems begin as soon as spectators try to fit all of the accidents and their consequences into some larger providential pattern. How, for example, would a providentially minded audience reconcile Ophelia's lot in life—her father accidentally killed when *Hamlet* lunges at what he thinks to be the King—with some larger, divinely ordained scheme?[58] What does that audience think when Ophelia's madness and subsequent suicide are transformed, quite disturbingly I think, in Gertrude's elegy which suggests that her death was an accident, the result of "an envious sliver" breaking as she climbed to hang coronet weeds over the river (4.7.148)?[59] Clearly there are contradictions in the providential reading of events in the play, and while these contradictions may not have risen to the level of spiritual crisis, they could have helped fuel the need for a more explicit providential vision in the conclusion.

Adding to this uneasiness would be the fact that both *Hamlet* and the guiding powers of "providence" begin to look like a trap when one begins to ask more precise questions about the providential outcome, and to some extent, the play itself encourages its audience to make this analogy. In almost every instance in which action is being "played" or arranged for an audience, that audience (Hamlet, Claudius) is a target of one sort or another. The sinister connotations of the art of contriving are enhanced, moreover, when that art is depicted as the right hand of "policy," a practice that reaches into affairs through the cunning use of what Polonius calls "indirections." While I think the play is ultimately trying to contrast this meddling form of "policy" with the more assured hand of God on events, the alignment of theatrical arranging with political plotting could not have been reassuring for the Christian spectator, even if a strict theological parsing of divine providence in the play could be employed to recast all of the agents onstage as the instruments of some higher power.

Ophelia, specifically, stands out as the subject of a particularly punishing form of providential manipulation, one that goes far deeper than

Polonius's paternal attempts to meddle in her affairs with Hamlet. If providential ideology works by drawing attention away from the world, Ophelia's "distraction" in act four looks like an almost permanent state of interruption—a pulling apart of consciousness so radical that regard can no longer return to consider events around her. In each of the scenes where she appears after her father's death, Ophelia is distinguished not simply by her disjointed speech and song but also by the fact that her attention can no longer be commanded by anyone on stage. Formulae such as "How now, Ophelia," or "How do you, pretty lady?" fail to recall her from this state, suggesting that attention has been entirely orphaned from the world without, however, being reattached to some otherworldly anchor.

The contrast of these scenes of "distraction" with Hamlet's calm before the rapier battle is startling, since both characters are really in parallel situations. Hamlet in act five and Ophelia in act four have both been drawn out of a previous state of attachment to the world by an accident, and both, in the wake of such a psychic detachment, are eventually drawn toward death.[60] Yet Hamlet faces death (or at least, the intimations of death) with an almost preternatural calm, using the occasion of "gain-giving as would perhaps trouble a woman" to reassert his own agency in accepting the challenge and carrying on with the game, regardless of its nature. While the difference in their demeanors does not, I think, show them to be essentially different in their response to the accident—each becomes radically distracted from the world in his or her own way—there is a gender asymmetry involved in their responses. Whereas Ophelia is depicted as the "patient" of such events, driven by the unexpected turn of events into an unspooling madness, Hamlet acquires a form of quasi-agency around accidents in the last scene, one that allows him to use these events as the occasion for revenge.[61] This qualified form of agency—a cooperation with divine providence which, paradoxically, allows him to fulfill the ghost's charge for revenge—completes a patrilineal circuit of obligation that a character like Ophelia is entirely excluded from. (Here, it is her brother that must take revenge for the death of Polonius.)

My reading of the play has now begun to fork off into contemporary concerns, since an Elizabethan audience would not have read *Hamlet* as an allegory for the psychic consequences of interpellation, or more broadly, for the mobile nature of theatrical consciousness. *Hamlet*'s allegories of spectatorship are worth dwelling on at the close, however, because they trump a certain myth of the theater that Shakespeare himself helped to generate: the idea that the theatrical experience is a dream made of wholly different stuff from lived experience, one in which the dreamer forgets that the "illusion" is not "real" and sinks into a world of untroubled "belief." *Hamlet* shows us why this could not be the case in the theater, and from its example we can surmise that such an untroubled state of belief did not await those who viewed life as a providential pageant either. To the extent that this mythology of belief and illusion still holds, we fail to grasp the ways in which theatrical action (whatever its ontological frame) is founded on the mobile consciousness of a distracted spectator, one who knows that his or her experience of events is contrived even if it seems to unfold of its own accord. If this fact is ever forgotten by that spectator, then theater forfeits its singular power to occupy a middle-state of action and becomes an odd form of spoken poetry, one which—like Beaumont's *Knight of the Burning Pestle*—might be interrupted at any moment when spectators decide they want to make improvements on what is said and done. Providence too, when deprived of the parallel expectation that the world has its own autonomous causes, becomes a swashbuckling story of direct divine action, a scenario that is hinted at in some of the more shrill providential literature which portrays God dispensing with accidents and striking down his enemies directly.

In recommending that we recognize the distracted form of spectatorship that accidents engage in the theater, however, I do not want to suggest that what I have been calling an attendant knowledge of artifice could be called out for inspection in any setting or, more important, that such a knowledge is ultimately a knowledge of the author's shaping power over his or her fictions. I have tried to avoid the suggestion that Shakespeare is doing the interrupting in *Hamlet*, but its persistence in my own reading of the play ought to confirm the fact that the theater in general, and Shakespearean theater in particular, are both institutions with their own hailing power. We can talk about *Hamlet*'s being interrupted, but not about its interrupter without reversing the terms of the early modern providential equation, conceiving of the author as a divinity who controls and foresees events as they unfold in a theatrical landscape. The idea that authors, rather than the desires and anxieties of a particular culture, are the guiding force in fiction is one with its own particular history. In acknowledging that history in our reception of the play, we have become distracted spectators of another sort.

CHAPTER 5

Accident and the Invention of Knowledge in Francis Bacon's Natural Philosophy

As a representative of the modern impulse to master nature and the techniques for understanding it, Francis Bacon would seem to have nothing to learn from chance and accident.[1] Like Niccolo Machiavelli who describes fortune as a woman who could be mastered through audacious action, Bacon consistently argues that nature—while liable to reveal some of her secrets by chance—must ultimately be commanded through a process of deliberate experimentation.[2] Indeed, a complacent reliance on chance and fortune for discovery in natural philosophy is one of the main targets of his reforms. In the *Novum organum* or *New Organon* published in 1620, for example, Bacon complains that

> [e]ven the works already invented owe their existence to casual experience more than to the sciences [*casui debenter et experientiae, magis quam scientiis*]; for the sciences we now have are nothing more than nice arrangements of things already discovered, not methods of discovery or pointers to new works.[3]

The sentiment expressed here and elsewhere—that natural philosophy cannot progress while languishing in the "fluctuations and meanderings of chance and rambling and disorderly experience" [*vel casus et experientiae vagae et inconditae undis et ambagibus*][4]—is meant to incite a desire for some more decisive and presumably masculine engagement with nature and its hidden processes. But the philosopher's experience of nature will have to become orderly if it is to become productive in the way Bacon foresees: without a method to put experience into such a conspicuous order, humans will never attain a practical mastery of natural processes.[5]

Readers of the *Novum organum* are told that this situation might eventually change. Here Bacon argues that if the method he proposes is adopted, the natural philosopher will be able to dispense with chance and take direct hold of nature through a knowledge of metaphysical

Forms. While these forms differ significantly from those described in Scholastic natural philosophy, the metaphysical determinants of natural processes in Bacon's system are no less universal in scope. In *The Advancement of Learning* (published 1605), for example, Bacon contrasts a merely physical knowledge of the world with the metaphysical knowledge of the Forms that he wants to acquire. We can think of the former as a circumstantial knowledge, one that can be applied only in familiar situations, while the latter has a nearly universal sweep of application:

> For Physic carrieth men in narrow and restrained ways, subject to many accidents of impediments, imitating the ordinary flexuous courses of nature, but "latae undique sunt sapientibus viae" [to the wise there are broad paths everywhere]: to sapience . . . there is ever a choice of means. For physical causes give light to new invention "in simili materia" [in similar matter]; but whosoever knoweth any form, knoweth the utmost possibility of superinducing that nature upon any variety of matter, and so is less restrained in operation. . . . The ways of sapience are not much liable either to particularity or to chance.[6]

As the last sentence suggests, Bacon believes that a philosopher's ability to manipulate nature is compromised whenever he has to rely on chance or particular circumstances for assistance. To the extent that chance participates in the invention or the use of knowledge, then, it would be impossible really to control natural processes in a deliberate, dependable way.[7]

Such passages confirm a rather traditional image of Bacon as modern hero or villain, a man bent on reversing the human dependence on chance and circumstance by expanding the frontiers of knowledge. Elsewhere, however, Bacon makes statements which suggest that he did not simply reject chance out of hand, at least not as a mode of inventing knowledge.[8] Consider the following passage from the *Novum organum*, in which occasion and chance are recognized as a source of discovery in natural philosophy, but then quickly left aside for a more deliberate approach. After cataloguing the Idols that stand in the way of philosophical progress, Bacon writes:

> So much then for dispelling despair and creating hope by the dismissal and correction of the errors of earlier times; now we must see what other grounds for hope there may be. This one comes to mind—if many useful discoveries have been made by some chance [*casu quodam*] or through some favourable circumstance [*per occasionem*], by men who were not looking for them and were engaged on some other matter, then no one can doubt that

much more would be discovered by men who were actively engaged in looking for them, and doing so in a methodical, not an impulsive or desultory way.[9]

A passage like this one shows Bacon's preference for method over wandering, a theme that develops consistently in his philosophical writings from 1603 through to his later pronouncements of 1620. But there is also a sense here that philosophers make real discoveries by chance, stumbling onto nature's subterranean secrets like a distracted stargazer stumbling into a well. While this is certainly not an ideal way of learning about the Forms, it is one way of learning about them. A better way would be to reproduce such "accidental" discoveries deliberately, something that Bacon believes possible only if experience is constrained by method. The real hope for knowledge, he writes in the *Novum organum*, lies in experience, "which if taken as it comes, is called accident [*casus*]; if it is deliberately sought, is called experiment [*experimentum*]."[10]

In what follows, I will present a less orthodox picture of Bacon's relationship to chance and accident, arguing that within his metaphysical system, accidents function like experiments when they reveal the Forms or their possible applications. While Bacon condemns accidental discovery as undependable, a theme that I will survey below, there is also in such condemnations a significant recognition that the Forms of nature become conspicuous only when the usual course of nature is abrogated. It will be important to understand why rare accidents have the power to reveal the Forms—what epistemological conditions allow them to serve as a means of discovery—and I will examine how Bacon understood these conditions. Once we see why accidents have been able to reveal what other modes of inquiry have not, we will be better able to understand how closely experiments resemble accidents in Bacon's metaphysical system. As I will argue, Bacon was not simply trying to eliminate accidental discovery from the philosopher's experience. Rather, he understood accidents as "experiments" made by chance—a rare convening of metaphysical Forms that reveals new ways in which those Forms can be combined. The Baconian program of experimentally vexing and artificially constraining nature, I will argue, can be understood as an appropriation or imitation of what nature (alone or with the help of a blind investigator) does spontaneously with the Forms in unusual circumstances. Such a program requires a relationship to chance and accident that is significantly more complex than the one suggested by the metaphor of mastering Fortune through audacious action. While this view of Bacon's program may force us to modify our understanding of his hostility toward chance and accident, such a reading is ultimately more consistent with his belief that knowledge of nature can appear only when nature is "vexed" or errs from its usual course.[11]

The Need for a Method

Bacon's complaint that past discoveries have all taken place by accident is almost habitual by the time he makes it in the *Novum organum*. As the title of his unpublished essay of 1603, *Temporis partus masculus,* or *The Masculine Birth of Time,* suggests, Bacon has already begun to identify chance as the implicitly feminine (because passive) form of progress in previous attempts to understand nature. Describing the alchemists, who have banded together to defend the views of Paracelsus against criticism, he writes:

> These men, in fact, formed a sort of confederacy to back up one another's lies. Thus they recklessly excited extravagant hopes, and if, in the course of their devious wanderings through the jungle of experience, they now and then lighted on something useful, this was by good luck rather than good guidance [*casu non ductu*].[12]

Later, after having attacked the views of Plato, Aristotle and Bernardus Telesius, Bacon admits that the Paracelsians are right in preferring experience to contemplation. But where does this preference lead them?

> A pig might print the letter A with its snout in the mud [*forte humi A literam impresserit*], but you would not on that account expect it to go on to compose a tragedy. That kind of truth which is deduced from scientific analogy [*ex scientiae analogia*] is very different from the mere intersection of the truth with some baseless hypothesis [*alia quae ex idoli sectione enuntiatur*]. The former is uniform and self-reproducing. The latter is contradictory and solitary. This holds good both for truth and works. If gunpowder had been discovered, not by chance (as they say) [*casu (ut loquuntur) et impactu*] but by good guidance [*ductu*], it would not have stood alone but been accompanied by a host of noble inventions of a kindred sort.[13]

Bacon gets polemical mileage out of the comic image of the pig, which here seems to resemble the monkey in the modern parable of probability who taps out some masterwork of literature at random.[14] Just as the letter drawn by accident [*forte*] cannot be punctually reproduced by the pig, so too the accidental discoveries of past natural philosophies have not resulted in subsequent discoveries. The discussion of accidental discovery, qualified though it is with the phrase *ut loquuntur,* which preserves the possibility that there is divine purpose in such discoveries, gives us a clear yardstick with which to measure the difference between the kind of knowledge Bacon wants (which comes *ex scientiae analogia*) and the kind that past inquirers into nature have accepted.

The condemnation of accidental progress in natural philosophy is even more strident in a text entitled *Cogitata et visa* (*Thoughts and Conclusions*), a work that Bacon composed during the years 1608–9 but did not publish. He begins with a declaration: "The discoveries men have up to now achieved cannot be credited to natural philosophy."[15] To what are they due, if not philosophy? Just before he makes this pronouncement, Bacon summarizes and then dismisses the meager accomplishments of medicine, alchemy, and the mechanical arts. All of these arts have disappointed, producing only a few discoveries at the cost of an enormous effort. Such efforts have nothing to do with the results obtained. Those discoveries can be attributed to "chance" [*casum*], he writes, which "without a doubt is a useful originator of things, but scatters her blessings on mankind only after tedious and tortuous wanderings [*longas ambages et circuitus donaria*]."[16] Clearly Bacon is trying to discredit previous attempts to understand nature by describing all such attempts as succeeding (only infrequently) by chance. But chance here also seems to be functioning as a mode of discovery, one that actually works, but which must be improved.

The kernel of value in the chance event seems to be the way in which it goes hand in hand with the unusual in experience. Thus in describing different modes of invention in the *Cogitata*—for example, dialectical invention and consulting past authorities—Bacon concludes with this last mode:

> Finally, there are inventions due to experience pure and simple. If it just happens, it is called chance [*casus*]; if it has been sought after, it is called experiment. . . . Those who try to discover the nature or mode of operation of anything by the repetition of random experiments [*multam et erraticam quandam experimentorum*] are never at one stay. They alternate between puzzled inaction or giddy activity; hot on the trail one moment, covered with confusion the next.[17]

There is an almost farcical way in which past natural philosophers have happened upon discoveries that they could not have possibly anticipated. Bacon is anxious, in fact, that these occasional successes may produce conviction in previous methods that instead should be abandoned. Leaving the need for reform aside for a moment, however, the fact remains that there have been discoveries made in natural philosophy and that these have been the result of an unusual disposition of circumstances which the investigator has not deliberately tried to arrange.

What we need to appreciate here is that while Bacon often complains that discoveries are made by chance, he also recognizes that chance discoveries are legitimate discoveries; in fact, they are the only ones that have been made so far. The problem with such discoveries is that they take a long time to turn up. Implicit in Bacon's statements about past discoveries is the belief that nature acting on its own, or the investigator wandering about in it blindly, can by chance approximate the conditions in which the Forms that govern nature become conspicuous.[18] Bacon's method, on the other hand, is designed to bring about deliberately those conditions that nature and ignorant investigators bring about spontaneously: a rare disposition of circumstances in which the metaphysical Forms recombine in unforeseen but useful ways. The key similarity between accidents and experiments is that both marshal the Forms in ways that the usual course of nature does not, and it is in this kind of "artificial" disposition or vexation of the Forms that Bacon places his hope for new knowledge. Before explaining how experiments produce artificially what accidents bring about spontaneously, I would like to describe in detail why Bacon felt that such unusual dispositions of circumstances could lead to a deeper understanding of how nature really works.

Disaggregated Forms and the Conditions of Their Discovery

A range of interpretive approaches has already been offered to explain Bacon's method of induction and its terminus: knowledge of the Forms, or *formae,* that govern natural processes in unalterable, lawlike fashion. For example, Bacon's Forms have been related to the *formae substantiales* of late Scholastic philosophy—formal elements that imparted, by a kind of internal efficient agency, certain attributes to bodies.[19] We also know that the operative power ascribed to the Forms, their ability to transform a given particular into a desired one, allows them to do the kind of work that alchemical and hermetic philosophers wanted to accomplish by other means.[20] These philosophical traditions thus seem to have influenced Bacon more than one might expect given his frequent criticisms of past approaches.[21] Certain legal modes of thought can also be adduced to explain Bacon's philosophical procedures of induction; for example, the process of finding axioms in induction has been compared to the determination of legal principles in case-law reasoning.[22] Studies like these have helped us to understand the historical sources of Bacon's thought. In the analysis below, however, I will be less interested in identifying the origins of Bacon's ideas than in explaining how his doctrine of the Forms allows the metaphysical determinants of natural processes to be revealed in unusual situations. It is this aspect of Bacon's doctrine, I will argue, that allows accidents to reveal—not an absence of regularity, as they did for Aristotle—but a hidden regularity that is concealed in the normal course of nature.

Bacon's inductive method has two strands, the one metaphysical and ideal, the other provisional and practical. As Lisa Jardine has pointed out, Bacon's natural philosophy aims at two distinct kinds of results: first, the fruits promised by the continued use of the *Novum organum* (knowledge of the *formae*) and second, benefits that will accrue more immediately with the aid of something called *Experientia Literata*, or "learned experience."[23] Learned experience is the more epistemologically modest approach to acquiring knowledge, on par with the kinds of probable knowledge (in the sense of "believable") that were being theorized in England during the seventeenth century.[24] Because knowledge of the *formae* would have to wait until an exhaustive collection of natural particulars had been completed, this more ad hoc approach aimed at discovering reliable conditions of operation within a limited but testable array of circumstances. Jardine describes this process as an improvisation of new experiments from old ones without the advantage of more general "axioms" from which new experiments or works could be devised. While the knowledge gained from this kind of experience would have limited application, it might serve as a down payment on the more globally applicable kind of knowledge that would come at the later stages of Bacon's instauration.

With *Experientia Literata*, one's knowledge and ability to act is still limited by the particular array of circumstances that he or she has already encountered in the world. The organon, on the other hand, will eliminate our reliance on *casus* to bring the relevant, light-bearing particulars into view for the enlargement of knowledge. In Book II, Bacon describes some of the basic terms of his new inductive logic, each of which is designed to represent certain correlations of metaphysical notions with physical properties that are invariant over the entire range of experiences one could ever have with nature. Natural bodies are "concrete natures" [*naturae concretae*], which are themselves composed of "simple natures" [*naturae simplices*] (yellowness, weight or ductility), each of which is always generated by a corresponding Form, or *forma*.[25] In gold, for example, one might identify the above natures but not know how each can be isolated or reproduced in other bodies. Assuming that one has identified what these natures are (itself a shaky assumption, Bacon will later admit), a set of trials can be devised in which the individual simple natures will be reliably correlated with the Forms that have generated them.

The correlation itself takes place by a process of elimination, so that those phenomenal features of a particular compound that are only circumstantially related to the presence of the Form itself can be excluded from its definition.[26] In the *Novum organum*, Bacon takes up the example of heat, which he has identified as a simple nature, and then he devises three tables of "Instances," or *Instantiae*: those in which heat is present; similar instances in which heat is absent; and finally instances in which heat is present to a greater or lesser degree.[27] From these tables an "induction," or *inductio,* is made, which involves the "rejection or exclusion" [*rejectio sive exclusiva*] of all the separate natures that are not found in any instance where the given nature is present.[28] Of course, this process of exclusion will not yield immediately conclusive results. Provisional "axioms" about the linkage between this simple nature and that Form have to be asserted in a "First Vintage," or *Vindemiatio prima,* an initial interpretation that is to be refined later by trials according to certain codified principles.[29] At times this "First Vintage" will be flawed, but Bacon feels it is more important to make such an interpretation than to give up at this point. "Since truth will emerge more readily from error than from confusion" [*quia citius emergit veritas ex errore quam ex confusione*], he writes, the understanding should be allowed to attempt an "interpretation of nature in the affirmative way."[30]

Telling the investigator to look for the Forms of simple natures accomplishes a great deal here, since now the task of the natural philosopher is not to account for "compound forms" such as lions or eagles—each of which would have its own unique purpose in the Aristotelian scheme—but instead to track the simple natures that compose those more obvious unities. The pursuit of such disaggregated *formae* represents a significant deviation from Aristotle's conception of purpose and form. In the words of one commentator:

> Baconian final causes, unlike Aristotelian final causes, do not presuppose the existence of immanent purposes in natural objects for the realization of complex "plans of structure." By the final cause of a characteristic of an organism or a feature of the universe as a whole, Bacon means the way in which it fits into the divine plan. Baconian final causes are related to substances in the same way as the purposes of an inventor are to his artifacts: They determine the way in which the artifact is constructed, but they are not the conditions which determine the way in which it operates.[31]

In this passage, Maxwell Primack points out a fundamental separation within Bacon's philosophy between the primary Forms—effective powers of determination with metaphysical scope—and the purposes that the Forms serve. Bacon does not argue, of course, that these primary Forms combine according to some atomistic chance. Certain preferred combinations are established in advance, during God's "six days' work," and so are sustained as the regular course of things. One's ability to appropriate the Forms for purposeful activity is not limited, however, to the regular combinations encountered in experience. The difference between divine and human creativity is not found in the ability to produce combinations of formal principles of determination, but the ability to establish that certain combinations will occur regularly. Thus in aphorism 5, Book II, he writes:

> For the principle of generating a single simple nature is the same as that of generating many, except that we are more hampered and restricted in dealing with several natures because of the difficulty of uniting so many, which do not readily combine, except in the natural and ordinary course of things. It has to be said, however, that this method of operation (that looks at simple natures, albeit in a concrete body) proceeds from those things that in Nature are immutable and eternal and universal, and opens up for human power broad paths, such as the comprehension of man (as things now stand) can scarcely grasp or imagine.[32]

Bacon's deviation from the Aristotelian scheme is of great consequence here. Whereas with Aristotle, any deviation from the regular course of nature had to be without a metaphysical cause and so could never become the object of purposeful human deliberation (all regularity being underwritten by metaphysically principled *per se* causes), Bacon's disaggregation of Aristotelian species forms into simple ones allows for the accidental deviation to be reproduced deliberately, because that rare deviation will have just as many formal determinants as any regular production. The only difference is in the combination of those determinants. With Bacon there are still accidental crossings of metaphysically independent lines of causation, as there were with Aristotle. But now new avenues for action are opened up when either chance or our own vexations of nature reveal other possible combinations of Forms, disaggregating the determined natures that might eventually be isolated for deliberate use.

The Transition from Accident to Experiment

Near the beginning of the second book of *The Advancement of Learning,* Bacon makes his famous division of the understanding into Memory, Imagination, and Reason, each of which corresponds to a field of learning—History, Poesy and Philosophy, respectively. Natural History, a subset of history in all its kinds, is itself divided into the history of nature in course, the history of nature erring or varying, and the history of nature altered or wrought (176). As some scholars have argued recently, this second category of nature erring is an important one for Bacon, allowing him to develop a category of natural occurrences that can be provisionally separated from explanatory theories or—in view of his desire to direct natural processes—an intermediate category between natural and artistic productions that will facilitate a swift transition from the wonders of nature to the wonders of art (177).[33]

Horst Brederkamp, in his discussion of European *Wunderkammern,* emphasizes the element of play that was associated with natural singularities—an element which Paula Findlen has also found in Italian collections of "jokes of nature" and curiosities.[34] "Play" here seems to imply an element of chance that is involved in the production of both nature's errors and related phenomena—for example, the stone that is cracked open to reveal the image of a landscape, or the perfectly rendered foam on the mouth of a dog, created accidentally when the artist throws a sponge at the canvas in exasperation.[35] Bacon too recognizes that there is an element of chance involved in the production of nature's errors when he urges the expansion of this branch of history:

> For I find no sufficient or competent collection of the works of nature which have a digression or deflexion from the ordinary course of generations, productions, and motions; whether they be the singularities of place and region, or the strange events of time and chance, or the effects of yet unknown properties, or the instances of exception to general kinds.[36] (176)

In keeping with the contemporary reading of such unusual instances as examples of nature's evolving or striving, we can read nature's *pretergenerationes* here as an intermediary stage in nature's "art," one in which chance and accident must be relied upon to produce effects that a more knowing artist (the natural philosopher) could eventually produce on command. But nature is not simply approximating the plastic arts here—although many did think of these marvels of nature as an expression of nature's formative power. Nature is also approximating experiment to the extent that it is bringing together the Forms in unusual, "artificial" ways. It is chance that creates these "artificial" conditions of revelation, just as the investigator will "artificially" dispose the conditions of nature's operation in an experiment.

For the twentieth-century reader, this relationship between chance and "artificiality" may seem unlikely, but to the Renaissance and early modern mind, the two were closely linked. While collections of curiosities could display nature's artifice in singularities that Aristotle would have said were produced by "chance," a parallel argument was being made in theories of art and painting. H. W. Janson has described the way in which the "image made by chance" was of particular interest to Renaissance artists, since in such instances nature seemed to display an artistic flair that the painter could imitate or contemplate for inspiration. Janson describes Piero di Cosimo staring at clouds and imagining that he sees pictures of equestrian battles and landscapes, much as Hamlet does when he shows Polonius a camel, weasel and whale in a cloud overhead.[37] Bacon himself reproduces one of the most famous loci in this neoclassical interest in relating chance and artifice. In describing the rare chance success of past natural philosophers, for example, which he compares to the success of a pig who accidentally draws the letter A in the dirt, Bacon is quoting directly from Cicero's *De divinatione*—one of the sources for Renaissance debates about whether chance could perfect art or merely imitate it.[38] If Bacon could see chance as infrequently imitating art, it is not surprising that he could see in the philosopher's art of induction a more reliable version of chance.

In Book II of the *Novum organum*, Bacon meditates on how the chance products of nature can be consulted in the process of induction to make individual forms show up more clearly. The Deviating Instances of nature, which result when the Forms fail to reach their goal in the process of combination, serve as a kind of tutorial in the powers of combinatory action that humans might eventually mimic in their own action upon nature. Such unusual effects may be more easily produced by humans than other unusual deviations in nature, since they show the dependence of Forms on the conditions in which they come together.[39] In such cases, Bacon writes, it will not be difficult to lead nature "back by art to the place where she chanced to go astray.... For errors on one side show and open up the way to errors and deviations on all sides."[40] The smooth transition from chance to art is obvious here, the spontaneous products of nature becoming signposts that point the investigator toward the Forms themselves. This is exactly what experiments are supposed to do in Bacon's system as well: make future "directions" for actions possible by turning up the hidden Forms that can then be employed at the investigator's will.

There are two other areas in which we can see Bacon associating chance with the revelation of natural processes. First we have Bacon's repeated assertions that ungoverned experience has brought important inventions to light when natural agents were disposed in unusual ways:

> Hence all the more noteworthy discoveries already made have, you will notice, been brought to light not by any small clarifications and extensions of arts, but wholly by chance [*sed omnino per casum*]. And nothing can forestall or anticipate [*repraesentat aut anticipat*] chance (which usually works its effects over long ages of time), except the discovery of forms [*inventionem formarum*].[41]

This notion of "anticipating" chance seems paradoxical until we recognize that induction is supposed to bring about methodically the kinds of unusual situations that chance can produce only occasionally. There is evidence in the *Novum organum* to suggest that Bacon thought his method would actually speed up the natural process by which time casually brings a useful invention to light. In a long aphorism from Book I, Bacon meditates on the way in which three inventions, the cannon, silk, and the compass, had to be discovered by chance because they could not have even been imagined before they were discovered. This advantage of chance—the way it "invents" despite the shortcomings of deliberation and imagination—is something that Bacon wants to reserve for his method as well. After describing the unprecedented nature of these discoveries, he says:

There is therefore every reason to hope that there are still many very useful things, which have not so far been discovered, hidden from us in the bosom of Nature, having no affinity or parallel with things already discovered, but quite off the beaten track of our imagination. No doubt they too will, at some future time, after many turnings and revolutions of the centuries, come forth, just as those earlier ones did; but with the method I am now discussing they can be expected soon, all together, and quickly.[42]

Bacon is aware that long periods of time are necessary for useful things to be "invented" spontaneously. The products of chance are by definition out of the ordinary—precisely what makes them useful in a world where the usual course of nature is unrevealing. Chance is thus not being repudiated when Bacon recommends experiment, but superseded by a more efficient mode of producing rare and unusual situations in nature.

Bacon also pairs chance with the production of knowledge about nature in his discussion of ancient myth in *De sapientia veterem* (*The Wisdom of the Ancients*), published in 1609. Benjamin Farrington, a commentator who has written about Bacon's work during the first decade of the seventeenth century, has remarked that this piece is similar to *The Advancement of Learning* in that it makes a measured public statement about matters that the philosopher has treated with far more polemical intensity in unpublished writings.[43] Spedding, Ellis and Heath did not include *De sapientia veterem* among Bacon's philosophical writings, but instead included it with Bacon's literary remains in their nineteenth-century edition of Bacon's *Complete Works*. Paolo Rossi, however, along with Fulton Anderson, has argued that in Bacon's allegorical interpretations of ancient myths, important statements are made about the philosophical system that he develops in manuscripts such as the *Cogitata et visa* and the *Redargutio philosophiarum*.[44]

Particularly noteworthy in this collection is Bacon's allegorical reading of fables surrounding Pan, fables in which he finds represented the "secrets" and "mysteries" of universal nature. At one point, he notes that

when Ceres, out of grief and indignation at the rape of Proserpina, had hid herself, and all the gods were earnestly engaged in seeking her out, and had dispersed several ways in search of her, it was Pan's good fortune to light upon and discover her by accident [*ex felicitate quadam contingisse*] while he was hunting.[45]

Later, after recounting and analyzing other features of the hoofed God, Bacon supplies a reading of this story that he believes contains the following "very true and wise admonition," namely:

that the discovery of things useful to life and the furniture of life, such as corn, is not to be looked for from the abstract philosophies, as it were the greater gods, no not though they devote their whole powers to that special end—but only from Pan; that is from sagacious experience and the universal knowledge of nature, which will often by a kind of accident [*casu quodam*], and as it were while engaged in hunting, stumble upon such discoveries.[46]

This image of the hunter ranging widely suggests that nature has a universal acquaintance with its own possibilities for action. Nature travels all paths, both the well-trodden ones and those little used, and when it moves along the latter, unusual discoveries are possible. Bacon is inspired by this mode of knowing, finding in the story of Pan a veiled description of how the natural philosopher must learn about nature. Like Pan, the natural philosopher should try to make discoveries by skillfully seeking out the hidden byways of nature.[47] The result: a natural philosopher so engaged will "by a kind of accident" [*casu quodam*] discover new modes of action that were previously unimaginable. Accident will have become an indirect form of action, a possibility suggested by the qualification of the term *casu* in the fable.

The hunt of Pan is a kind of shortcut to new works that Bacon elsewhere associates with Learned Experience [*Experientia Literata*].[48] While induction "invents" new experiments by consulting general axioms about how different natures are generated, Learned Experience tries to find unusual instances of those natures by the "method of experimenting" [*Modus Experimentandi*].[49] Bacon describes several techniques for turning up these unusual instances—what he calls the Variation, Production, Translation, Inversion, Compulsion, Application, Conjunction, and the Chances of Experiment. On the one hand these techniques are designed to lead the investigator to new arrangements of circumstances or objects that he or she may not have been ready to imagine unassisted. Like the topics of rhetorical invention, these *topoi* of Learned Experience spur the investigator on to what may be remote to his or her experience (or memory), but which might usefully be consulted. On the other hand, the "method of experimenting" seems designed to take advantage of the way in which virtual "experiments" are produced by chance in experience. While describing the "Translation of experiment," for example, Bacon shows how several artificial techniques—for example, the cider-maker's practice of leaving fruit to ripen in bunches—are actually a way of "imitating" something useful that happens by chance in nature.[50]

One is not restricted to imitating or translating the chances one finds, however, as most arts have been in the past.[51] Bacon's last topos, the Chances of Experiment [*Sortes Experimenti*], encourages the investigator to imitate chance itself rather than particular instances of its action. This means trying whatever outlandish thing one can imagine, since

> [t]his form of experimenting is merely irrational and as it were mad, when you have a mind to try something, not because reason or some other experiment leads you to it, but simply because such a thing has never been attempted before. Yet I know not but in this very process (of which we are now treating) some great thing may be involved; the leaving (I say) of no stone in nature unturned. For the *magnalia* of nature generally lie out of the common roads and beaten paths, so that the very absurdity of the thing may sometimes prove of service. But if reason go along with it; that is, if it be evident that an experiment of this nature has never been tried, and yet there is great reason why it should be tried; then it is one of the best ways, and plainly shakes out the folds of nature.[52]

In a sense, all experiments are meant to shake out the folds of nature in this way, disposing circumstances in a manner never before tried. But chance has a privileged place in this mode of invention, since it is the principal means by which these unusual arrangements have been secured in the past. Experimenting for Bacon is an imitation of what chance does, folding or unfolding different parts of nature in ways that jostle the imagination and the usual disposition of things. Until a knowledge of Forms allows the philosopher to anticipate all of what chance might do—leaving experiment behind for a life of action—the natural philosopher will have to stage more artificial "chances" or "accidents" in order to bring that knowledge closer.

Accident, Experiment, and the Situational Limits of Knowledge

There are at least two fundamental similarities between accident and experiment in Bacon's natural philosophy: both are a result of an unusual disposition of circumstances, and both are understood to be a more "artificial" version of what nature does when left to its own habits. Although there is clearly an important difference between these two—experiment is a deliberate process, while "accidents" like the discovery of gunpowder or nature's deviating instances come about by chance—Bacon thought of these as different versions of the same process. Accident and experiment are cousins in Bacon's system, two ways of bringing about an unusual situation in which knowledge can be acquired. This attentiveness to the situational constraints on knowledge is raised to the level of a philosophical virtue in his philosophical works, one that survives in the practices of experimental philosophers later in the seventeenth century. Boyle's experiments with the air-pump are a particularly well known example of knowledge being produced in an "artificial" situation—the (putative) vacuum in his glass globe serving to mark off a space in which knowledge could be legitimately produced.[53] As Boyle remarked about his own experimental practice, one cannot trust "obvious experiments" because they exhibit phenomena that may proceed from more than one cause; when such a plurality of possible causes exists, "a more artificial trial may determine, which of them is true."[54] The irony of course, both in Bacon's natural philosophy and the experimental philosophy that follows, is that such "artificial" situations tell the philosopher more about nature than nature in its usual state.

Bacon's interest in what Hans Blumenberg has called the "systematization of accident" should force us to rethink the relationship of his experimental method to the sensibilities that might have inspired it.[55] Both politically and intellectually, Bacon was writing at a time when one's first reaction to the obvious was to treat it as a form of deception. The famous Cartesian scheme of doubting received ideas and impressions is a Continental example of this distrust, but we can find similar sentiments expressed in Bacon's work as well.[56] Consider the following statement from the *Novum organum:*

And just as in ordinary life the true personality of a person and his hidden thoughts and motives show themselves more clearly when he is under stress than at other times, so things in Nature that are hidden reveal themselves more readily under the vexations of art than when they follow their own course.[57]

We can think of Bacon's attempt to put stress on nature, in part, as a means of wrenching evidence from what is essentially a reluctant witness.[58] On this reading, skepticism about the reliability of knowledge is relinquished once a sufficient amount of force has been applied to the object of study.

This analogy of the deceiving witness, however, does not fully capture Bacon's sense that the mind itself, as well as the world, is working to keep the philosopher in the dark. There are idiosyncrasies of the individual, of culture and of language that might flush knowledge back into its hiding place when the philosopher is near. In such a situation, accidents—events that no one can either suspect or manipulate—acquire significant epistemological power. This recognition of the role of accidents in breaching secrecy was already present in the rhetorical tradition, for example in Cicero's argument that the plots of conspirators could be exposed, often irrefutably, by chance interruptions.[59] While such interruptions were often a prominent feature in early modern plays dealing with secret plots, they also found their way into contemporary "intelligence" reports, suggesting that providence—acting through a network of spies—might sometimes "interrupt" the schemes of those conspiring against the crown.[60] Given this tendency to view accidental events as occasions on which the veil of deception might be drawn aside, we can understand why Bacon might have viewed accidents as an interruption in the otherwise concealing regime of nature. In a world of secrets, be they secrets of nature or secrets of state, accidental knowledge could sometimes be credible knowledge.

But we should also understand the provisional favor shown to accidents in Bacon's work in light of a lively Renaissance interest in the role of chance in social and political life. The *Book of the Courtier*, for example, reminds the reader that the most easy and nonchalant gestures are those that must be the best practiced.[61] One would thus be a fool to assume that what appeared to be a casual meeting in the piazza, or an "accidental" revelation of passion might not have been staged precisely to deceive. Conversely, a rhetorical interest in occasion or *kairos* made many aware of how the right circumstances could complement the speaker's art when they were recognized and acted upon.[62] Finally, the notion of Fortune as an abstract force opposing deliberate human action dominated humanist writings on prudence, virtue and *ingenium*. As Machiavelli writes in *The Prince*, Fortune is "mistress of one half of our actions" — a conservative estimate, given his tendency elsewhere to resign all outcomes of human affairs to Fortune's inscrutable power.[63] While these developments in contemporary intellectual and political life are not usually associated with experiment, I believe that they help us to understand Bacon's sensitivity to situation, circumstance and the artifice of "accident" in the production of natural knowledge.

The arguments I have made here suggest a broader continuity between a "situational" sensibility that informed rhetorical and political culture in the sixteenth and seventeenth centuries and Bacon's belief that one had to get control of circumstances for nature really to be understood. By situational sensibility, I mean the awareness that what one knew or could do was limited by the disposition of circumstances at a given moment. Within this sensibility, there was a special place for accidents, since they were moments when circumstances had been spontaneously gathered into a new and unusual pattern. To the extent that this arrangement made unprecedented actions or insights possible, accident could be counted upon to outsmart even the most deep-seated habits of the mind of clinging only to what it knew already. Like the skeptic's doubt, accident could be cultivated in order to dispel erroneous or habitual interpretations of nature. Bacon's pairing of the accident and experiment may also help us relate the experimental tradition of the seventeenth century to treatments of chance and accident in the ancient and medieval tradition. There is a significant break with that tradition when Bacon argues that accidents — which happen rarely and unexpectedly — can reveal something that is otherwise hidden in nature.[64] But when Bacon turns to chance and accident as examples of the kind of unusual circumstances to be reproduced in an "experiment," he has more than one thousand years of vigorous speculation on what chance and accident are to work with. Perhaps the accidental event continues its illustrious philosophical career into and out of the seventeenth century, not just as a calamity in the world or a topos in debates about God's providence but also, more figuratively, as something to be sought out "indoors" — in the artificial conditions of the laboratory. While such unprecedented events can no longer be called accidents once they are produced deliberately, there is no reason for us to forget that the spontaneous version of these rare events had a past philosophical life in ancient and medieval thought.

Bacon was well aware of the way in which Fortune, chance and accident might assist the inquirer in the search for knowledge, but he was like Machiavelli in wanting to beat Fortune at her own game. The systematic attempt to "vex" nature in experiment was designed to put an end to dependence on lucky accidents as a principle of inventing natural knowledge and, by extension, to eliminate philosophy's debt to the feminine "births of time" in which accident was the ascendant mode of discovery. But if we see this move as a banishing of Fortune and chance from the experience of the natural philosopher—or in more grand terms, as the triumph of a modern, masculine will to control the uncertainties of experience—we overlook a more subtle dependence on contingency in his philosophical program, one that is rarely avowed in the confident rhetoric of advancement which pervades Bacon's work. Bacon is indeed attempting to beat Fortune at her own game, but his rhetoric of domination is contradicted by the real debt that he owes to chance and Fortune as the tutors of discovery. Like Machiavelli, who recognized that one must sometimes submit to Fortune in order to master her, Bacon's logic of discovery suggests that he too saw the necessity of submission, which meant taking on some of Fortune's conventional feminine qualities in order to gain the upper hand.[65] The point for Bacon was not to banish accident, but to exceed it in experiment, and in doing so to harness its revealing powers. Without a doubt, this process of vigorous experimentation was meant to culminate in a modern capacity for autonomous self-assertion. Most immediately, however, it involved becoming as variable and improbable as Fortune herself.

CHAPTER 6

Wonders Taken for Signs: The Blackfriars Accident of 1623

"What chaos? What fearfull objects? What lamentable representations?" These are the words of the Protestant minister Thomas Goad, penned after listening to a harrowing eyewitness account of the Blackfriars accident from John Gee, a preacher from Lancashire who had joined the auditors in the three-story garret house that collapsed on October 25, 1623. Gee had been brought to Lambeth so that the archbishop of Canterbury and his chaplain Goad could hear a firsthand account of the disaster, which was about to ignite a sectarian pamphlet war throughout the city. According to Gee's description of the accident, a sudden break in the floor plunged those who had gone to see the Catholic speaker that day into a calamitous heap of "rubbish and dead carcases." Spectators rushed to the scene where Gee—"beyond my owne expectation and humane understanding"—emerged and began searching the wreckage for survivors. As people arrived from different quarters of the city, some to taunt and throw rocks at the Catholic victims, constables shut the precinct gates to prevent rioting. It was only with the assistance of another Protestant minister, William Gouge (whose lecture at the nearby Blackfriars church was interrupted by the terrible noise), that Gee and a few other "men of good understanding" were identified and shuttled out of the precinct so that their testimony could be heard by the archbishop and his chaplains.[1]

Thomas Goad heard the makings of a great narrative that day. He would waste no time collecting several such versions of events into a rendition of his own entitled *The dolefule even-song*. Goad was not alone in wanting to rehearse the particulars of this astonishing event, which was recorded in state papers, diaries, and an array of songs and religious pamphlets. Like Goad's pamphlet, almost every account underscored the narrative quality of the event, suggesting that the effect of Blackfriars was that of seeing life become drama, or perhaps, of recognizing that the world of lived experience was theatrical from the start. The structural analogy between a providential world and the stage, so exhaustively explored two decades earlier in *Hamlet*, could thus be made in the opposite direction. Even someone learning about the accident secondhand could be inspired to declare the scene a fearful "representation," particularly in a situation like this one in which human prudence and foresight had been so suddenly upended by disaster.

In proposing that the two terms in the analogy between world and stage were reversible, however, early modern providentialists assimilated two very different kinds of order that were increasingly kept apart over the course of the seventeenth century. On the one hand, the providential interpretation of historical accidents appealed to an order that governed the natural world, one that was created by God and maintained either actively or passively through his care. While this order was the object of theologies of providence, it was also quite clearly the province of natural philosophy, which treated the action of mundane or "secondary" causes. Providential interpretation also, on the other hand, invoked the kind of order that was manifest in poetic fictions, an order founded on imaginative acts rather than the predictable behavior of bodies or substances. Whereas in fictions the "causes" of events might best be described as suppositional—such "causes" existed on the presumption that they advanced some requirement of the fable—the causes of accidents in the world could be assigned to the autonomous power of nature, the human will, or God himself. When readers of Goad's pamphlet wondered at the providential irony of Blackfriars, then, they were applying assumptions about the nature of order in poetic "fictions" to a world which, according to both the traditional Aristotelian natural philosophy and the emerging experimental one, could be explained with reference to secondary causes alone.

Given the emphasis in early modern poetic theory on the didactic nature of most acts of "poesy," it is not surprising that a strong moral strain could be found running through the discourse of the world.[2] When judged according to the pre-Kantian aesthetic canons of the seventeenth century, even the most brutal manifestations of God's revenge on sinners could express a certain poetic order, however divisive and punishing that order might seem.[3] If we are willing to follow the providentialists' lead in saying that there was a poetics of God's providential action in "accidental" wonders, however, we need to ask how the awed response that Aristotle associated with tragic catastrophe was transformed when it was experienced by a worldly spectator. Could assumptions about the nature of theatrical order be harmonized with existing and emerging knowledge about how the natural world worked? Did it matter that many of the portents, marvels and providential accidents that were so exciting to early modern readers were just as responsive to nonpoetic, nonhermeneutic modes of explanation during this period? How would a poetic wonder at God's divine purpose change once the events that expressed it were explained in causal terms?

There were no simple answers to these questions, in part because the relationship between divine purposes and natural causes was itself changing in the early modern period. Recent historical work on wonders, marvels and prodigies suggests that during the seventeenth century, naturalistic explanations of unusual phenomena and events were becoming increasingly dissociated from interpretations of them as signs of God's judgment or of future disasters.[4] Whereas a century earlier, for example, a cloud that resembled a chariot might have heralded God's displeasure with the earthly church or an imminent battle, natural philosophers in the seventeenth century would have been more careful to invoke only natural causes to explain such a striking occurrence. But if learned writers came to prefer secondary causes in their analysis of wonders, this did not mean that naturalistic interpretations of these events completely eclipsed the providential or supernatural ones that took wonders for signs. As Lorraine Daston and Katharine Park have argued, portentous explanations of wonders like monstrous births persisted throughout the fractious seventeenth century in England, just as they had on the Continent during the wars of religion.[5]

What changed during the sixteenth and seventeenth centuries was not the kinds of causes (natural or supernatural) that could be assigned to strange phenomena, but rather the kind of divine purpose or intention these phenomena were understood to express. Among natural philosophers, the potential for divergent and so disruptive interpretations of the meaning of wonders led them to eschew open speculation on the value of wonders as signs as the seventeenth century progressed. Unwilling to mix the two modes of explanation, Francis Bacon created an interpretive division in his *Advancement of Learning* whereby the sober insights of natural philosophy could be carefully partitioned from the interpretive flights of divine speculation. Efficient, material and (with certain modifications) formal causes would be the province of natural philosophy and metaphysics, whereas final causes—while they were of interest to the metaphysician—would ultimately be the business of the theologian.[6] By the end of the seventeenth century, a mild disgust for the portentous interpretation of wonders would be the hallmark of intellectual responsibility among natural philosophers such as Robert Boyle, even if providential interpretation of certain kinds of wonders persisted in other quarters.

In principle, however, causal analysis and the poetic interpretation of "signs" were not mutually exclusive modes of explanation. Secondary causes could be understood to cooperate with divine wishes in order to create some significant but wholly natural production in the sublunary sphere. The case of monstrous births was perhaps the most conspicuous area in which cooperation could be discerned. Such cooperation could be understood as an "accidental" convergence of secondary causes, an idea that was used both by theologians and by natural philosophers to account for the creation of "preternatural" effects from natural processes.[7] Such a subtle form of overlapping or divine "indirection" assumed a different logic of divine control than that which governed the activist conception of God's miraculous intervention. When wonders were understood to have miraculous and so unique causes, their startling appearance could be taken as evidence that they communicated a similarly unique, divine purpose. Miraculous explanations of wonders thus assumed that the divine significance of unusual phenomena was guaranteed by the kind, rather than the configuration, of causes that produced them. It was just this form of isolated miraculous action which Calvin and other Protestant theologians would reject on the grounds that miracles were being used by the Catholic church to lead Christians into error.[8] Bacon too would resist miraculous occurrences in his natural philosophy on theoretical grounds, although in fact it was difficult to distinguish the true miracle from an occurrence with a natural cause working to odd effect.[9]

When we turn to a historical accident such as the Blackfriars disaster of 1623, we are faced with a wonder whose natural causes were never seriously doubted, but whose meaning as a sign remained irresistible to those who wanted to explain it. Precisely because it was an accident in the Aristotelian sense, Blackfriars complicated the distinction between poetic interpretation and causal analysis that would have been more clear cut in cases of direct divine intervention, like a voice issuing from a burning bush. In surveying the competing narratives of the disaster in detail below, I want to foreground some of the ways in which accounts of Blackfriars invoked particular narrative and dramatic canons in order to give the accident some deeper meaning, a rhetorical strategy that was repeated in a range of wonder pamphlets published in the first decades of the seventeenth century. If sectarian debate about Blackfriars was about meaning, however, it was also quite clearly about natural causes and their linkages to divine intentions. The stake in this battle of words was the power to assert some precise relationship between those causes and purposes—the power to shape or impose a poetics of God's worldly action on the world by dramatizing that action in narrative form.

The story I have to tell in this final chapter is thus one in which narrative descriptions of wondrous events imply a particular understanding about how meaning is produced in and through the world, first by God, and then by those who must interpret his will in his "actions." The focal point of the story is not so much the theories of God's providence that were called on to explain various "accidental" occurrences as it is the particular affective states that gripped the individuals who witnessed or read about those events. Such feelings or "passions" were nearly identical with the fear and awe associated with tragic wonder, and so it seems crucial to link them historically with the narrative conventions which produced them. But those passions are crossed, in the historical accident, with wonder of a philosophical sort, a feeling that was often understood to anticipate knowledge in advance of its possession. The affective response to Blackfriars—and by extension, a whole range of early modern accidents that did not literally take place on stage—is thus a mingled form of tragic awe and philosophical curiosity, one which deserves a name of its own.

Early modern philosophers and theologians inherited a longstanding tradition of thinking about wonder as a response to some novel situation or object, the result of a lack of understanding that invited further engagement. The idea that the affective state of wonder could itself be explained as an effect of ignorance was a classical one: Aristotle held that wonder in the face of the unexpected was the spur to learning.[10] Augustine, too, when he considered the awe-inspiring qualities of the world, suggested that spectacular events manifest a fundamental human ignorance of the causes at work in creation. Because all causes are ultimately an expression of God's incomparable creative power, he writes in *De civitate Dei,* they should be a perpetual source of amazement.[11] When this definition of wonder as cognitive lack met with the growing conviction that marvels had natural causes, wonder at unusual events seemed destined to be replaced by knowledge of the causes of those events.[12] Francis Bacon worked to institutionalize this transition from wondering to knowing in England—a move that his medieval predecessor Nicole Oresme had already begun to lay the groundwork for—by recommending that unusual natural productions be included in natural histories.[13] The feeling of wonder was also becoming susceptible to physiological-dialectical analysis. In his *Passions of the Soul*, published in 1649, René Descartes defined wonder as a "sudden surprise of the soul which brings it to consider with attention the objects that seem to it unusual and extraordinary."[14] Significant for Descartes is the element of surprise, so that wonder becomes a passionate form of considering or regarding something that precedes any knowledge of how that thing ought to be understood.

For learned writers of the seventeenth century, wonder becomes a passionate departure with an intellectual destination.[15] The cause of that reaction, when wonder is cast in the Aristotelian, cognitive framework, seems to be both the rarity of certain occurrences and an individual's ignorance of the causes that brought them about. There was another kind of wonder, however, that could be felt toward unexpected events during this period, one which was increased rather than dampened by a knowledge of natural causes. This kind of wonder is a response to the disposition of agents in the world rather than their extraordinary power, a reaction that takes place because an accident has shifted the spectator's attention from the mundane causes of the event, freeing it instead to gather meaning from the circumstances in which the event took place. This final process of interpretation puts an end to wonder, supplying a vacuum that natural explanation cannot fill by introducing a more subtle force which can shape events without suspending the natural processes at work in the world.

I would characterize the awed apprehension of a deeper meaning in the accident as an anagogic wonder that concerns spiritual meaning, one which is opposed to the cognitive kind of wonder that seeks out missing causes. As the characteristic early modern response to seeing the parallel realms of drama and lived experience converge, anagogic wonder implied a unity or interconnectedness among all elements in the created universe, a unity whose pattern and significance exhausted the explanatory registers of necessary or probable causation.[16] This almost mystical unity of purpose was traditionally associated with Scripture by medieval exegetes—it was one of four levels of meaning (along with the literal, allegorical, tropological) that could be identified and pursued by the reader of God's word. In reviving this term, I want to suggest some crossover between assumptions about the hermeneutic unity of Scripture and the anagogic unity of a providentially ordered world. The textual nature of such assumptions are implicit in Northrop Frye's use of the term in *The Anatomy of Criticism,* in which he proposes that anagogic interpretation implies "a universe in which everything is potentially identical with everything else."[17]

Instead of making it the counterpart of a cosmos structured along textual lines, however, I would characterize anagogic wonder as a historical phenomenon related to the prominence of the theater as metaphor for the signifying capacities of the world. As I will try to demonstrate below, anagogic wonder was not at odds with the sense that natural causes could be found for marvels, since coincidences and accidental events did not require a miraculous suspension of natural causes. Indeed, what was wondrous about accidents in the world was the way in which they could accommodate a mode of providential speculation that was wholly indifferent to the demystifying powers of naturalistic explanation. To the extent that anagogic wonder held these two different interpretive impulses in tension without allowing one to cancel another, it fostered a particularly mobile form of ideological consciousness that could be integrated into both the religious and philosophical currents of the period.

The Blackfriars Accident

As he explained what had happened in Blackfriars to the archbishop, John Gee probably had reason to be anxious. The group of nearly three hundred auditors who had assembled in the gallery adjoining Hunsdon House that afternoon was predominantly Catholic, and Gee's presence at such a gathering suggested (as he confessed to the Archbishop) that he was wavering in his Protestant faith.[18] Rarely had so many "Papists" ventured to gather in such an open public meeting, and while the assembly was hardly a secret, the Catholic evensong may have seemed like an open provocation to Protestants who were on the lookout for Catholic activity. Published accounts of the accident itself tend to be quite detailed in their descriptions of what happened that day. After the audience had been ushered up a stairway into the chamber, Robert Drury apparently entered the room in a red cap and white linen robes. An hourglass was set up to keep track of the time, a detail that in hindsight would suggest the crowd's imminent encounter with mortality. Mounting a chair in order to address the crowd, Drury lectured on the parable of the man who is not prosecuted for a debt but then prosecutes another for the same offense. After he had finished discussing the parable, one pamphleteer writes, Drury raised his eyes up toward heaven and began to pray.

The crack of breaking beams and falling timber was loud enough to be heard throughout the Blackfriars district. Along with Drury himself, nearly one hundred people fell to their deaths, breaking first through the top floor and then again the one below. A few survivors huddled in a small corner of the room, which had now all but caved in; these were described as "spectators" of the grim "scaene" below who could escape only by digging their way through the adjoining plaster wall. (An illustration of the event, taken from Richard Horde's Latin elegy, *Black-Fryers*, appears on the cover of this book.)[19] The sudden "downfall" of a building during a Catholic sermon seemed an open invitation to interpret the event providentially, either as a specific kind of divine vengeance against practicing Catholics or as a herald calling members of both faiths to personal account. The outpouring of contempt for dead or dying Catholics on the scene was so intense that many Protestant pamphleteers subsequently urged readers to consider the disaster in a spirit of charity and reverence. Well before trained theologians got their chance to interpret it, however, Blackfriars seems to have ignited sectarian passions and prompted individuals to interpret civic life as the scene in some didactic stage drama.

Indeed, when the Blackfriars accident occurred, a range of religious convictions could be expressed in narratives that didactically rehearsed details of the accident in one way or another. Four accounts of the catastrophe were published in 1623 alone, each referring to the downfall of the floor in a Blackfriars garret house as an "accident"—lamentable, fearful, memorable or fatal, depending on the writer. The first account to appear in print was Goad's *The dolefull even-song*, a pamphlet which advertised itself as a "particular and impartial narration" of a "lamentable accident" that was both sudden and fearful.[20] Goad's claim to impartiality seems to rest with his own reluctance to pass judgment on those who died or were injured, a task that he says is best left to the reader. Ample guidance is provided, however, for those who are uncertain about what the event might mean. Halfway through his story, Goad urges survivors to "lay it to their hearts, whether this sudden stroake and cracke be not the hand, and voice of God, to call them home from wandering after forraine teachers."[21] The accident here becomes a call that should turn both Catholics and wavering Protestants away from their errant journey through foreign pastures. While the nature of the call should be immediately recognizable, Goad seems aware of the fact that the accident must be seen from a certain perspective for its specific providential meaning to appear.

For Goad and the other pamphleteers who interpreted this event, an empirical explanation for the accident could exist alongside the providential interpretation of what happened. After the floor fell through, Goad describes how an official inquiry into the catastrophe found the most "probable apparent cause" of the downfall to be a fragile support beam forced to bear too much weight. This detail about the weakness of the floor support was a standard feature in many published accounts of the accident, crucial because rumors were circulating that Protestants had sawed through the floor beams in an attempt to sabotage the meeting. John Wilson even managed to fit the point into a song about the event that was published anonymously in 1626:

> For plaine it was, in strictest view,
> That by the peoples presse
> And sommeyrs mortazing undue,
> They came to distress.[22]

Yet while a natural cause for the accident could easily be given, there was still something to be explained. For Goad and others who recognized a possible empirical explanation, the significant *explanandum* was not the structural weakness of the building, but the fact that the accident happened to these people (predominantly Catholics), during a particular activity (listening to a Catholic sermon) and on a particular date (November 5 by the Gregorian calendar)—the same date as the Catholic gunpowder plot.

What needed to be explained about the Blackfriars accident was not the weakness of the floor supports but the specific circumstances that brought together so many people in a shaky building for a Catholic evensong. Even a child could see that the circumstances were meaningful in this instance, and to illustrate the point, Goad tells the story mentioned in the Introduction about a ten-year-old girl who responds to the accident by saying that the downfall would cause a public scandal for the religion of those involved.[23] An anonymous account of the accident published soon after it happened raises the question of circumstances explicitly. The writer of the book, *Something written by occasion of that fatall and memorable accident in the Blacke Friers on Sonday,* argues that the accident expresses God's vengeance against Catholics for assembling, urging readers to "plainly denuntiate what God threatens, and manifestly confirme Gods judgements against them, when he determines a vengeance."[24] The "wonder of the judgement" consists both of the number of people killed with so little means and the fact "that it must fall out on the 5. of their November" (12). While "the Papists will have it a meere accident," the reader is told, "and so impute it to the Antiquity of the building, and the rottonnesse of the timber" (9), it still remains to be explained why Drury's auditors were set up in that particular unhappy place to hear the sermon. Why, the writer asks, should Catholics describe the victims of the catastrophe as if they were martyrs? Were they forced to go into these rooms to die? The description of the event as a "meere accident" overlooks precisely what needs to be explained, namely the particular disposition of circumstances that allowed for the event to happen as it did.[25] The answer to these questions cannot be supplied through causal analysis, but must be given as a narrative.

When writers begin to ask these kinds of questions, we see that the Blackfriars accident elicited some of the same passions and interpretive impulses that dramatic accidents occurring on stage would have provoked. Indeed, several of the writers who describe the downfall recognize that the accident produced wonder, pity and admiration in those who had either witnessed the event or heard about it indirectly. The anonymous author of a book entitled *The fatall vesper* writes that the sound of the fall and cries of the injured roused many to come and "see this wonderfull event, and this object so full of admiration." Later he urges Londoners, Protestants and Papists all to "repent for by these wonderfull signes and tokens, it doth appeare most clearely that the kingdome of heaven is at hand."[26] It seems as though the sheer quantity of human suffering, along with the fact that there was really no natural cause that explained why these people chose precisely the wrong place to assemble, provokes a mixture of fear and awe in those who confront the event, a reaction this writer tries to contain by suggesting a specifically dramatic meaning to the occurrence.[27]

Of all those who published accounts of the Blackfriars accident in

1623, the anonymous author of *The fatall vesper* is the most self-conscious about the dramatic nature of the event. Making what to most would be an obvious analogy, the author writes that the world is "a Theater, and the actions thereof a continued Scene whereby our Lord hath manifested unto us these designes of his impartiall judgments" (C1v). When viewed in this dramatic context, the circumstances of Drury's death can be mined for their tragic pathos. Notice how the astonishing destructiveness of the catastrophe is transformed into sympathy for Drury—and so also, the Catholic plight—in the following passage:

All the day before, which was the last that ever his eyes beheld, he was observed to be wondrous sad and pensive, contrary unto his wonted humour and disposition, he being a man of a free, merry, and affable conversation, as though that some spirit of prediction had foretold him of that fatall disaster, which was at hand. Thus we reade of Caesar, that hee was possessed with a strange and unwonted sadnesse that morning when he entred into the Senate house where he was stabbed to death by the Senators. (C3r)

Later we learn that a gentlewoman of a noble house approached Drury before he entered the room, warning him of the "unfitness" and "uncapacitie" of the place—clearly a reference to the inherent weakness of the building. Drury ignored the warning, and "being led on by a divine and fatall necessitie, which blinds the judgement of the wise men of this world, hee told her that hee did meane as then to preach" (C4r). When represented in this way, Drury's sudden death seems less a punishment than a noble kind of sacrifice, a quality that led some to suspect that the piece was written by a Catholic sympathizer.[28]

An explicitly pro-Catholic version of events was published by John Floyd, although he too was unwilling to put his name to the story he had to tell. The title of his book, *A word of comfort. Or a discourse concerning the late lamentable accident of the fall of a roome, at a Catholike sermon, in the Black-friars at London*, suggests the palliative nature of the work.[29] Like the author of *The fatall vesper*, Floyd notices the link between the circumstances surrounding accidents and the wonder they produce. As Floyd surveys the long history of accidents that have befallen Christians in the past, often in circumstances that suggested Christians were being punished, he attempts to dampen the particular force of this occurrence by making such accidents the ordinary course of the world. For example, Floyd points out that "in respect of the circumstance of the tyme," the "wonderfull destruction" of the city of Nicea was a scandal to the early Christians (20). He goes on to explain that just as Valence, the Arian emperor, began to persecute the Nicene faith, the city of Nicea was destroyed by the worst earthquake in memory. In Floyd's words, the circumstances seemed arranged

> as if God togeather with the Emperour, heaven togeather with earth had co[n]spired agaynst the Nicene doctrine, of Christs being Coeternall and Consubstantiall unto God his Father. (20–21)

When Floyd goes on to chastise "[t]hese our Antagonists that are so jolly and jocund, so puffed up with pride at the fall of a rotten chamber upon some few at a Catholike sermo[n]" (21), he criticizes the tendency to give circumstantial interpretations of accidents befalling certain groups. In fact, it is these interpretations and not the fatal consequences of accidents that must be regularly suffered by Catholics. Floyd writes that there is no greater affliction to God's servants than "the happening of strange & dreadfull mischances, that carry a shew of his anger agaynst their Religion, wherby the enemies therof harden their soules as stone, agaynst it" (5). Subtly, then, Floyd's book shifts the point at issue. Whether or not the death of Catholic auditors was a punishment sent by God, the cause of that accident was "vulgar and ordinary," which makes the exploitation of that accident for persecutory purposes so much more oppressive from the Catholic point of view.[30] Once this kind of mean-spirited overinterpretation of accidents is identified as the problem, Floyd can cite a range of similar calamities that have befallen Catholic Christians in the past in order to begin consoling his readers. The end result should be the cessation of wonder, a passion that Floyd views as tempting even Catholic believers to accept the punitive interpretation of the accident offered by their antagonists. Floyd writes:

> [W]hy doth Heresy insult upon Religion, in regard of an accident common unto men, and unto which their owne sect is continually subject? . . . Why doth Fayth complayne or wonder at this course of Gods provide[n]ce which he has set down to himselfe in his Word, and which hath been still his ordinary since the world? (6)

Clearly Floyd and others who tried to explain this event to the reading public were aware of the rhetorical life this accident would have—a life that depended on the possibility of there being more than one way of interpreting the event. No one setting out to write such an account could have been dull to these possibilities and, as a consequence, the need to shape perspective where perspective was so crucial.

The Blackfriars accident is not simply an early modern lesson in perspectivism, however. The event also demonstrates how little it mattered that a natural cause could be found for what had happened. What was astonishing about the accident was not the miraculous nature of its causes, but the way in which independent, well-understood processes could be seen working together to produce a disaster of astonishing proportions. It was this convergence of a specific group of people in a particularly infelicitous place that provoked wonder or astonishment, and the task of those interpreting the event was either to excite or dampen those reactions in ways which built on the evidence of surrounding circumstances.

Blackfriars and "Accident" Literature: 1600–1623

While learned accounts of marvels tended to be more philosophically precise about their potential causes, treatments of marvels meant for a popular audience tended to mix terms like "wonder," "accident," "chance" and "miracle" in ways that defy systematic treatment. The accounts of the Blackfriars accident that I have discussed above were clearly intended for a wide audience of London readers, but they are unusual in their attempts to specify precisely the kinds of causes that might have contributed to the accident.[31] In particular, the attempt to distinguish between "mere accidents" and providential ones attests both to the intensity of the sectarian interests which were brought to bear on the event and the susceptibility of this kind of disaster to multiple, but not incompatible, modes of explanation.

As we have already seen in Chapter 4, a popular literature of sorts was developing during the late sixteenth and early seventeenth centuries that recorded unusual or noteworthy "accidents" for the information or edification of those who wanted to read about them. Writers who produced these "accident" pamphlets or collections were not so much trying to convey a precise philosophical concept when they used this Latinate word as they were attempting to frame the stories they had to tell in an intellectually respectable way. Referring to an event as an "accident" distanced what was about to be described from both the immediate causes that brought it about and the interests of those who might have a stake in interpreting it. One way to understand the early modern use of this word is to think of how the word "incident" is used today, often in legalistic or scientistic narrations of events that are known to have some significance, but which must be referred to outside of their putative causes or meanings in the initial stages of representation.

Accounts of the Blackfriars accident belong to this larger genre, not simply because of their subject but also their manner of representing the circumstances surrounding the catastrophe.[32] The sense that "accidents" might have some deeper spiritual meaning—particularly those that suddenly and unexpectedly overtook the people who suffered them—was already being cultivated in the literature that chronicled God's providential "judgments" several decades before Floyd and Goad wrote their accounts in 1623. As I argued in Chapter 4, these accounts tended to emphasize the value of "wonderful" accidents as spectacles that should be "regarded" for their edifying message. An anonymous pamphlet entitled *Lamentable newes out of Monmouthsire in Wales* (1607), for example, describes the "wonderfull and most fearefull accidents of the great overflowing of waters," telling readers that "howsoever natural causes, as Gods instruments doe claim their partes in them, yet they proceed from the Lords own direction, who by his punishing of others with them, doth threaten grievous calamities, even against our vice."[33] In addition to emphasizing the providential meaning of these events, however, the popular literature often recognizes the role of chance and accident in bringing such punishments or deliverances about. An account of floods occurring during the same year as the one cited above describes how different regions are chastised by the rising waters "according to the quality and proportion of . . . offences."[34]

One of the examples given is of the "miraculous" delivery of a man who, seeing the waters rising, returns home to save his wife and children. Recognizing that all of his possessions are going to be engulfed, he attaches a "Bore of Writings" to a rafter in hopes that it will be found after the flood, thus allowing him to prove his property holdings once the floodwaters have receded. Meanwhile, the water rises and carries the family away so that "the Husband & the wife lost one another: the children and Parents were parted: the Gentleman in this whirle-wind of waves, being forcd from his hold, got to a beame, sat upon that . . . til at length encountring with the side of a hill . . . there he crept up" (C2r). While the husband is weeping on the hill at the "Tragedy of his deere Wife, and deerest Children," he spies the bore of writings that are floating toward him. Retrieving these, he is "myraculously" delivered from the ordeal with both his own life and property. This and other unlikely deliverances that take place during the flood are described as "Tragicomicall Scaenes [which] have beene acted upon this large Stage of waters" (C3r). What is striking about this particular story is the way in which the coincidence of the "bore" returning to the man and the romance trope of the family separated in a shipwreck support a specifically tragic or tragicomic reading of what has happened. The word miracle seems hyperbolic in this context, but the sense that coincidences are what warrant an ironic, providential reading of these scenes—facilitating, in the end, a more pointed fear of divine retribution—is clear from the circumstances that the author has chosen to include in the narration.

Another example of the accidental deliverance at sea appears in a short pamphlet entitled *Lamentable newes, shewing the wonderfull deliverance of Maister Edmond Pet sayler* . . . (1613).[35] The narrator describes how Master Pet was coming from Newcastle with a fully laden ship when a storm struck, forcing all those aboard to abandon the vessel. While Pet encouraged the men on board to pray for God's mercy, the entire crew was drowned in the midst of supplication—all but Pet, who

> after he had bene under water, by Gods helpe tooke hold of the maine Mast and got out his knife and cut certaine cords or lines and made shift to get up to the top of the Mast, and there tied himselfe, for, feare least by the strength of the winde and rain he should be blowne off into the Sea. (A2v–A3r)

Floating on this mast, Pet is at the mercy of the sea for a day and a night. When a ship arrives within sight, however, those on board are too busy to rescue him. (The narrator makes an explicit comparison to the biblical story of the good Samaritan here.) Two days later, we learn, "there came towards him by Gods appoyntment a man of warre . . . who did shew him kindnes and mercy" (A3r). The crew eventually drop Pet off at a port and when Pet is finally reunited with his wife, she cannot recognize him because he is so swelled and weather beaten. As with most providential literature of this kind, readers are instructed how to interpret the example given in this man's experience:

> And see and heare and give God praise, yet more of Gods wonderfull kindnes in delivering this Maister Pet once before, who comming from a farre voyage in a Ship of Marchandise, by misfortune the Ship was split, the Ship and all the goods lost, and to the number of eighteene persons drowned.

And this man left alive to tell unto the world what God had done for him, that all that heare it might praise the Lord. (A3r–A3v)

This story of mercantile disaster at sea is topically related to some of the dramatic and philosophical stories I have analyzed elsewhere. Egeon's rescue in *The Comedy of Errors*, for example, might be one fictional predecessor of this particular account. Of related interest here is also Francis Bacon's critique of the painting of shipwreck survivors in the *Novum organum*. Such an image, he objects, is misleadingly offered as evidence that God saves all those who call on him.[36] This kind of interpretation—clearly of a piece with the one offered in *Lamentable newes*—is misleading, Bacon goes on to say, because those who pray and are drowned never survive to be painted. The substance of this objection is that one should not cite a cause for the man's rescue (Pet's virtue) that cannot be uniformly applied to others in the same situation (that is, Pet's drowned, praying shipmates).

In this didactic history of Master Pet, the word "fortune" is used even when it is at odds, doctrinally, with the providential thrust of the narrative. Like many popular accounts of such events, the terms are chosen for their descriptive value or the generic canons (romance, tragedy) that they engage. Most important in the context of the argument I am trying to advance, however, is the way in which the accidental or "fortunate" nature of Pet's rescue contributes to the writer's sense of wonder at the event. Clearly there is nothing miraculous about a ship's spotting a floating man, nor of a storm's sinking a ship. What requires providential interpretation of Pet's survival (indeed, what sanctions the use of poetic conventions in recounting an otherwise factual event) is the sheer arbitrariness of the forces that first endanger and then ultimately save the man from death. Presumably, readers will respond both to the event and to the conventions used to represent it with the kind of wonder appropriate to similar "meaningful" accidents found in poetic fictions.

Another kind of "accident" that was associated with misfortune or mischance during this period was fire, no doubt because of its proverbial volatility.[37] Accounts of individual fires, while a huge genre in their own right, can nevertheless be included under the rubric of popular accident literature. In 1621, for example, a pamphlet entitled *Newes from France* describes the "great losses which happened by the lamentable accident of fire in the citie of Paris." Included in the account of the disaster is a description of the parliamentary decree that was made after the disaster, "to prevent the like mischance in time to come."[38] Clearly the fire could be interpreted in two ways, either from the standpoint of its providential meaning or its empirical causes, and the former did not rule out the latter. As the author explains, the providential purpose of the accident is to rouse sinners who must

> turne unto him, who is the Soveraigne Ruler.... Then (I say) he employeth the great forces of the heavens, and the Elements, thereby to heale the ulcer of their vices.... Which plainely appeareth by the deplorable accident happened of late in the Citie of *Paris*, where the force and furie of fire strucke such an astonishment in all the inhabitants, that they thought the Towne, like a second *Sodome*, would suddenly have been consumed to ashes. (A2r–v)

While the providential meaning here is clear, the author's willingness to call fire an "element" and recognize its place in the heavens (that is, lightning) suggests that God's judgment here is being exercised through, not in spite of, the natural processes that he or she is familiar with. On the one hand, we are given a fatalistic and somewhat melodramatic rendering of the event in passages like this: "Divers servants ... induring and feeling the rigor of that mischance, stood in the like manner as others did, ready to pay their debt to cruell destiny" (A3r). Apparently servants could be punished by such accidents as well, even if they had no stake in the property loss. The author is also interested in the material conditions that allowed the fire to catch and the official reaction to the catastrophe. At one point, readers are told how the fire spread from the Merchant's Bridge to surrounding houses "by meanes of certaine beames that lay crosse over one to another" (A3r). Later, the king's attorney general is given a commission "to make information of the beginning of that fire, considering the divers reports that were spred abroad in the Towne, that might bee a meanes to procure great trouble in the same" (Bv). The immediate political concern here is that without any official determination of the natural cause for the event, rumor mongers may exploit the ambiguity of the event to stir up civil unrest.

The last wondrous event I want to discuss, also associated with fire, is described in a pamphlet published in 1622 entitled *A relation of the most lamentable burning of the cittie of Corke* ...[39] The pamphlet is a followup to one published previously that year recounting a battle in the sky between "certaine birdes, called Stares, or Starlings" near the city of

Cork. Apparently, in October of the previous year, a large group of these birds divided into what seemed like two camps and then initiated a battle in the sky, "which was so strange and admirable an accident . . . the like hath very seldome or never bin heard of."[40] While it is clearly the unprecedented nature of the starling battle that evokes wonder here, the event that follows it confirms—by a strange coincidence—that the portentous interpretation of the initial event was correct. On the last day of that same month, a sudden darkness filled the sky:

> Inhabitants stood thus wondering at the extraordinary darkenes, suddenly they heard a terrible clappe of thunder; And at the same instant they saw a dreadfull lightning, with flames of fire breake out of the Cloudes, and fall upon the Cittie at the same instant, at the East end, and the highest part of the Cittie. At that very place where the Stares beganne their Battell, and where they first fell downe, being killed in the fight. (4)

The phrase "at that very place," of course, is meant to suggest that the fire which destroyed the city and the unusual starling battle are purposefully related. This is the kind of purpose which is expressed through coincidences, however, not simply rare or unusual occurrences.

Like so many other accident accounts, *A relation* emphasizes the way in which such events should move individuals to "considerations of Repentance." What is unusual about this sequence of pamphlets is that they superimpose two kinds of wonder. The first kind—which is a startled reaction to the unprecedented battle in the sky—is supposed to initiate a process of introspection and, ultimately, spiritual reform. Failing to heed the sign, however, itself becomes a sin that is then punished by another natural occurrence of remarkable destructive power (a lightning strike):

> The Battell of Birds over the Cittie being so strange and wonderfull an accident, might have moved them to considerations of Repentance, but they sleighted it over; And now they find (which others may feare) it is good to lay hold on Mercy whilest it is offered. (9)

The "poetic" justice that links the two wonders is itself a source of wonder here, although this time the response is described as a kind of fear. Presumably the reader will feel this fear as well, but only if a certain kind of passion is stirred up by the coincidence of the lightning strike occurring at the "very place" of the bird battle. As with the other accounts of providential "accidents," this relation of events is calculated to produce wonder at the deeper meaning behind events that are both rare and contain an element of chance or coincidence. A single phrase may be all that is required to suggest that element, so that what first appears causally unmotivated can then be ironically inverted in a providential interpretation. Although this response—of wondering and inverting—may not lead to the more precise distinction-making and reflection that a philosopher would recommend, the kind of anagogic wonder which the popular "accident" literature evokes seems nonetheless to accommodate whatever probabilistic or naturalistic explanations can be offered for the events being described.

Anagogic Wonder: A Situational Passion

Several years after the accident at Blackfriars, William Gouge (who found Gee in the rubble and brought him to Lambeth) published a treatise on God's providence to which he appended a sermon he had preached about the catastrophe a week after it happened.[41] The sermon is of a piece with other anti-Catholic interpretations of the event, urging listeners to see "the finger of God" in the circumstances surrounding the collapse of the building. The treatise, however, has more general things to say about how people should respond to signs of God's activity in the world. In *Gods three arrows*, Gouge complains that divine judgments are "not regarded, but are passed over without any right observation of them" (105). He recommends instead that "Gods judgements are duly to be observed. Of them saith the Lord, Behold, regard, and wonder marvellously" (104). Gouge's point here is not a new one as far as this kind of admonishing literature is concerned. Wonder in the face of an accident like the one that happened at Blackfriars marks the moment when an individual's attention or "regard" is suddenly detached from the concerns of this world and turned elsewhere. If we understand wonder in this way, the affective response to accidental events becomes the inner complement of a communal, sectarian impulse to "see God's finger" in events happening in the world. Public pressure and inner passion work together in this process to assimilate the individual into a providential scheme on occasions that are beyond anyone's power to expect or predict. As I have tried to show above, the fact that this kind of wonder was not blunted by the natural causes that could be found for accidental events would make this mode of ideological assimilation quite durable. Until accidents stopped happening, there would always be the potential for wonder at accidents and the deeper significance that could be found in them.

In making anagogic wonder a point of entrée into the spiritual order, I want specifically to avoid the implication that a learned eagerness to find natural causes for wondrous events could insulate the individual from this process of assimilation. Because purpose is grasped in the mundane coincidence with extraordinary effects, no explanation of such an event through secondary causes would really be sufficient to empty it of its spiritual purposes. Rather, those purposes would persist in the face of natural explanation, entangling those who recognized them in the (logically prior) assumption that the world was structured along the same lines as a theatrical fiction. One did not need to start with this assumption; it could be deduced later from the experience of anagogic wonder itself, or simply recalled with the help of someone who was spiritually further along. But if the experience of anagogic wonder implies a certain familiarity with the doctrine of providence, it is also connected to a particularly theatrical brand of early modern consciousness whose sources and determinants are not strictly theological. Anagogic wonder would not have been as powerful if there had not been a steady flow of plays, political treatises and popular wonder literature asserting the fundamental similarity between the created world and a theatrical fiction, an analogy whose explanatory value had reached the level of common sense, or even a cliché, around the turn of the seventeenth century. The popularity of accident literature as a print genre, even the popularity of particular accidents like the one that occurred in Blackfriars, ensured that both the theatrical metaphor and the responses it enabled would be absorbed by a large cross-section of the reading public.[42]

Because it is so closely linked with this theatrical cast of mind, anagogic wonder is best understood as a passion with cultural rather than transcendental conditions of possibility. Some of these conditions would persist throughout the seventeenth century, for example the widespread belief in divine providence; the sense that natural processes (no matter how inscrutable or regular) were nevertheless capable of producing unforeseen outcomes; a willingness to see in the accidental disposition and arrangement of things a particular kind of artifice or order. Of course, accidents themselves would persist as well, particularly in a city like London that continued to bustle and grow at an astonishing rate throughout the seventeenth century. The stage, however, would slowly begin to lose its value as the representative "scene" in which the spatial patterns of human action were played and therefore understood. Over the course of the eighteenth century, fictional accidents would take up residence in the private space of the novelistic imagination, a space in which events "occurred" or unfolded at the leading edge of a constant verbal flow instead of the bounded *platea* of the theater. We can think for a moment here of Robinson Crusoe, carefully relating the circumstances of his encounters with Providence on the island, all of which have been anticipated by the spiritually reformed author who is telling the story retrospectively.[43] This type of narrative structure, while it is not necessarily representative of the novel as a genre, nevertheless suggests how the novel's representation of accidents will focus on their effects on an evolving consciousness rather than on their role in revealing some hidden order in the world. In this respect at least, the cultural life of anagogic wonder—linked as it was to a spatial calculus of justice and order—would be limited by its dependence on the theater as a metaphor for the nature of experience.

A growing hostility toward purposive forms of explanation within natural philosophy would further limit the intellectual and cultural prospects of anagogic wonder. As the seventeenth century progressed, learned writers would increasingly avoid the intermixing of purposive and naturalistic forms of explanation—precisely the kind of mixing that had allowed natural causes and divine purposes to fuse into a powerful, anagogic unity earlier in the century. As a result, anagogic wonder would be delivered to the regions of poetic or religious imagination, regions that were understood to stand apart from the emerging experimental spaces of English natural philosophy. We see an early example of this philosophical trend in Francis Bacon, who is reluctant to probe unusual occurrences in nature for their hidden providential meaning. In addition to prohibiting appeals to final causes in his natural philosophy, Bacon argues that providence itself may be beyond human powers of explanation. Like a potentate who uses his obedient subjects for a purpose they cannot guess, he writes in *The Advancement of Learning*, God acts in "politique" ways that are so subtle they cannot be appreciated by the individual observer.[44] For Bacon, the appropriate place for these providential interpretations is in poetical fictions or Feigned History, genres in which the imagination is allowed to embroider events with more justice and divine retribution than is apparent in experience. The use of Feigned History, he writes:

hath been to give some shadow of satisfaction to the mind of man in those points wherein the nature of things doth deny it. . . . Therefore, because the acts or events of true history have not that magnitude which satisfieth the mind of man, poesy feigneth acts and events greater and more heroical; because true history propoundeth the successes and issues of actions not so agreeable to the merits of virtue and vice, therefore poesy feigns them more just in retribution, and more according to revealed providence.[45]

While Bacon does suggest elsewhere that providential justice is occasionally revealed in mundane events, in general he is reluctant to give individuals free reign in interpreting these events.[46] This reluctance would appear again in the writings of Thomas Sprat, the apologist for the Royal Society who recommends attending to "experiments" rather than Providences. Writing after the Interregnum, Sprat argues that given the present temper of "our Nation," "[t]his wild amuzing mens minds, with Prodigies, and conceits of Providences, has been one of the most considerable causes of those spiritual distractions, of which our Country has long bin the Theater."[47] Once again providential interpretation is described in terms of drama, suggesting that the analogy between world and theater was still pervasive enough to merit an active condemnation.[48] Spiritual consciousness within this theater, moreover, is described as a form of "distraction" that must be remedied by a more sober form of philosophical discipline: experimental natural philosophy becomes for Sprat—as perhaps it had been for Bacon—an alternative technique for managing attention, for keeping it contained in a productive, interested way.

Yet while the Blackfriars disaster illustrates the manifold ways in which unusual accidents piqued the early modern theological imagination, learned skepticism of the Baconian sort would not have been enough to discourage the furious speculation that followed such an event. Writers like Gouge and Goad did not have to do much in order to make something out of the accident: what was striking about it was that a great many dramatic conventions were already "there" in what happened. The real ideological power of this and other accidents in the sixteenth and seventeenth centuries lay not in the interpretations that could be attached to them but in the almost automatic way in which they shifted assumptions from the theatrical or poetic realm into the experiential one. If such a transposition—thinking of the world as stage or plotted fiction—was a commonplace of Renaissance culture, it seems nevertheless to have been the event itself rather than the overeager mind of a religious zealot that occasioned the analogy. A large body of Protestant doctrine on providence might make such a literalization of the theatrical metaphor seem obvious or even obligatory, but the Blackfriars accident suggests that something other than doctrinal assumptions made Londoners receptive to the competing explanations that were being offered.

For providence to assign a divine cause to the purposes that appear spontaneously in the world, there has first to be an individual who feels that something needs explaining. Anagogic wonder is a name for this feeling, and in early seventeenth-century England, the Protestant doctrine of providence supplies a more or less systematic set of underlying assumptions that such a passion anticipates.[49] In a sense, anagogic wonder destines the individual to unearth these providential assumptions in the same way that cognitive wonder steers the natural philosopher down the path toward knowledge.[50] But this is true only in a sense. Wonder need not always lead to knowledge or a communally sanctioned set of assumptions, even if the inevitability of both can be retroactively located in the passion that led to them. Anagogic wonder, at its most paradoxical, is an early modern passion in the future perfect, one that will have been the consequence of whatever "providential" assumptions are found to explain it. What is important about anagogic wonder is thus not just the sectarian views it engages but also the movement it implies—from the natural world to a poetic fiction, from explanation to interpretation, from a precipitous inference back to its enabling assumptions—in the wake of a passion rising from within.

Epilogue

Once John Gee had been pulled from the rubble of Blackfriars, his response to the accident was to meditate almost obsessively on the fact that the persons to his left and right perished while he was inexplicably "saved." In the vocabulary of anagogy explored in the last chapter, Gee had experienced what William St. Thierry once described as the *osculum aeternitatis,* or "kiss of eternity"—a sense of the transcendent that had been transferred from the realm of Scripture to encompass the particulars of the world itself. This reaction is one of several that I have argued were characteristic of the early modern engagement with accidental events. Alongside Gee's response we could set Bacon's philosophical appropriation of accidents into his program for experiment, or Shakespeare's use of accidents as a hallmark of theatrical "indirection." For each of these early modern writers, accidents illustrate the power of circumstances to accomplish the unforeseen, a power that is grounded in the specifics of a unique time and place but that can nevertheless be understood to serve some deliberate purpose or "end."

My own approach in this study has been to foreground the artifice of accident, although I have assumed that these events were themselves artifacts of a particular culture rather than some theatrical divinity. Certainly, however, I have borrowed some of the interpretive assumptions of the writers I study, foremost among them the idea that circumstances ought to be consulted when trying to understand a cultural phenomenon, here the early modern experience of the accidental. This habit of looking to particulars and circumstances for some larger pattern is a hallmark of interpretive historicism, which is what I see myself practicing in this study of accidents across a number of discursive frames. Only by looking at the culturewide dissemination of the trope of accident can we understand what these events might have "meant" to those who wrote about them at a particular time. Taking this horizontal view of a particular cultural moment is not the same thing as providing a structural analysis of how accident works as a rhetorical device or a general account of its possibility as an "idea." Clearly accidents can be illuminated by these kinds of analysis, and I have relied on them myself at times. But the integrated picture is more revealing, even if it is acquired through the willful juxtaposition of autonomous cultural forces into an interested whole. Such interested wholes are by definition the object of a culturally aware historicist criticism, regardless of the names—"ideology," "culture" or "discourse"—that are found to describe them.

Perhaps, then, there is some secular form of anagogic interpretation that always arrives to suffuse a cultural moment with hermeneutic meaning for the distant interpreter. In offering such an interpretation, I do not feel obliged to experience the "kiss of eternity" as the providentialists might have done. Nor do I feel compelled to unearth some Pynchonesque conspiracy of historical actors, as if developments in the past could be the effect of some deliberate, global plan. Even in using terms like "ideology" or "culture," which I have found indispensable, I have tried to avoid the view that certain interpretations of "the accidents of experience" were controlled by some interested individual or group. Such a view voids the power of cultural explanation by undercutting its collective basis, substituting a quasi-divine agency or "man behind the curtain" for what is more properly a convergence of interests on a particular event or moment. But I do experience some form of affective alteration in my encounters with the past, one that grows out of the apprehension of pattern and connection in elements which are not linked by some immediate, universally acting cause. Perhaps this experience of the particular and the contingent is the starting point for cultural criticism, providing a crucial form of resistance that goads the interpretive impulse into action. That interpretive impulse resembles the literary impulse to read the unity of meaning in a text: it even has some of the hallmarks of providential interpretation. But by emphasizing the particularity of a cultural moment over the logic of an idea or origin, an interpretive historicism can grasp the situational sources of meaning in a given culture without locating that meaning in an individual subject or transcendental structure.

Although I have stopped short of offering a causal explanation for the turn toward accidents in the late sixteenth and early seventeenth centuries, I believe such a turn was conditioned by several interrelated historical developments discussed throughout this study, for example the arrival of new theological ideas about God's providential action, the prominence of the stage as a metaphor for experience and the rise of a philosophy of nature that valued the particular as a means of arriving at the universal. The story I have told about the rising interest in accidents could be integrated into other narratives as well, for example that of the rise of an urban commercial culture (which required deliberately "accidental" meetings for exchange) or the diffusion of religious ideas in popular print. These latter two developments have stood, perhaps, too far in the background of my study, but in giving them less prominence than they deserve, I hope nevertheless to have gained a more precise sense of the specific narrative processes and intellectual displacements that allowed the accident to become an avenue of revelation during this period. None of the larger cultural developments or individual writers I have examined here could have single-handedly thrust the accident into prominence, and so no genetic account of its emergence as a cultural phenomenon can be exhaustive. But clearly there was an ensemble of conditions—I am tempted to say convergence of circumstances—that made early modern writers particularly alive to the philosophical, narrative and affective possibilities posed by accidents at the turn of the seventeenth century, and those conditions were both material and imaginative.

If the accident serves as the occasion on which a will to interpretation is brought to bear on a contingent past, then the early modern fascination with accidents reveals something more general about historicist interpretations of cultural particulars. Seeing this analogy between interpreting accidents and interpreting cultural artifacts is one of the most interesting consequences of having tried to understand these events as an object of narrative practice and historical change. It is an analogy that I only slowly became aware of as I worked on the topic—collecting examples of accidental events and writing about them in different contextual frames—but in the end it is the one I find the most intriguing. Like accidents, the particulars of the past can be apprehended only indirectly, as objects of interpretation. But like accidents, cultural particulars can be significant only to someone who imagines that circumstances might have been otherwise and are meaningful because they were not. Such an imaginative capacity belongs as much to those who lived within a culture of accidents four hundred years ago as it does to those who interpret it now.

Notes

Notes

Introduction

1. See Stephen Greenblatt, *Marvelous Possessions: The Wonder of the New World* (Chicago: University of Chicago Press, 1991); Steven Mullaney, "Strange Things, Gross Terms, Curious Customs: The Rehearsal of Cultures in the Late Renaissance," in *Representing the English Renaissance*, ed. Stephen Greenblatt (Berkeley: University of California Press, 1988), 65–92; Lorraine Daston and Katharine Park, *Wonders and the Order of Nature: 1150–1750* (New York: Zone Books, 1998); Paula Findlen, *Possessing Nature: Museums, Collecting, and Scientific Culture in Early Modern Italy* (Berkeley: University of California Press, 1994); Krzysztof Pomian, *Collectors and Curiosities: Paris and Venice, 1500–1800* [1987], trans. Elizabeth Wiles-Portier (Cambridge: Polity Press, 1990); Philip Fisher, "The Poetics of Wonder," in *Meaning and the Visual Arts: Views from the Outside*, ed. Irving Lavin (Princeton: Institute for Advanced Study, 1995), 175–93. A survey of these developments appears in Carolyn Walker Bynum, "Presidential Address: Wonder," *American Historical Review* (February 1997): 1–26.

2. The emphasis on wonder as a passion rather than simply an object has been adopted by Daston and Park in their latest study, *Wonders and the Order of Nature*. The literary power of this particular passion has been explored by Greenblatt in *Marvelous Possessions* and more specifically in "Resonance and Wonder," in *Learning to Curse: Essays in Early Modern Culture* (New York: Routledge, 1992), 161–83. Earlier critics interested in the literary structures that produce wonder include Tzvetan Todorov, *The Fantastic: A Structural Approach to a Literary Genre* (Ithaca: Cornell University Press, 1975); J. V. Cunningham, *Woe or Wonder: The Emotional Effect of Shakespearean Tragedy* (Denver: University of Denver Press, 1951); and Baxter Hathaway, *Marvels and Commonplaces: Renaissance Literary Criticism* (New York: Random House, 1968). On the awed response to certain theatrical displays of political power, see Stephen Greenblatt, *Renaissance Self-Fashioning: From More to Shakespeare* (Chicago: University of Chicago Press, 1984), ch. 2; Stephen Orgel, *The Illusion of Power: Political Theater in the English Renaissance* (Berkeley: University of California Press, 1975); and Mullaney, 68–73. On the theatrical metaphor in early modern religious experience, see William Bouwsma, *John Calvin: A Sixteenth-Century Portrait* (Oxford: Oxford University Press, 1989), ch. 11; Anne Blair, *The Theater of Nature: Jean Bodin and Renaissance Science* (Princeton: Princeton University Press, 1997), ch.

5; and Ernst Robert Curtius's history of the analogy between world and stage in *European Literature and the Latin Middle Ages*, trans. Willard R. Trask (New York: Pantheon Books, 1953), 138–44.

3. On the linkage of Baconian experimental science with the early modern interest in wonders, see Lorraine Daston, "Marvelous Facts and Miraculous Evidence in Early Modern Europe, *Critical Inquiry* 18 (1991): 93–124; "Baconian Facts, Academic Civility, and the Prehistory of Objectivity," in *Annals of Scholarship* 8, no. 3–4 (1991): 337–63; Katharine Park and Lorraine Daston, "Unnatural Conceptions: The Study of Monsters in Sixteenth- and Seventeenth-Century France and England," *Past and Present* 92 (1981), 20–54; and William Eamon, *Science and the Secrets of Nature: Books of Secrets in Medieval and Early Modern Culture* (Princeton: Princeton University Press, 1994), 299.

4. There have been studies of *Fortuna* during the period, for example by Aby Warburg, but the topic of "accidental events" themselves has largely been left aside in Anglo-American scholarship. Recent interest in the topic of contingency among German-speaking scholars has led to some important work in this area, however. See the special issue "Kontingenz" of *Poetik und Hermeneutik* 17 (1998); Walter Haug and Burghart Wachinger, eds., *Fortuna* (Tübingen: M. Niemeyer, 1995); and Klaus Reichert, *Fortuna oder die Beständigkeit des Wechsels* (Frankfurt: Suhrkamp, 1985).

5. As the text of the *Poetics* becomes available to European readers in the second half of the sixteenth century, the wondrous becomes increasingly viewed as one of the privileged effects of poetics and rhetoric. See Cunningham, *Woe or Wonder*, ch. 4; and James V. Mirollo, "The Aesthetics of the Marvelous: The Wondrous Work of Art in a Wondrous World," in *The Age of the Marvelous*, ed. Joy Kenseth (Hanover: Dartmouth University Press, 1991).

6. Aristotle, *Poet*. 1452a1–11. See Aristotle, *The Complete Works of Aristotle*, ed. Jonathan Barnes, vol. 2 (Princeton: Princeton University Press, 1984), 2323.

7. See, for example, Keith Thomas's *Religion and the Decline of Magic* (New York: Charles Scribner's Sons, 1971), in which he points out that a common theme in post-Reformation theology was "the denial of the very possibility of chance or accident" (79). See also Paul H. Kocher, *Science and Religion in Elizabethan England* (San Marino: The Huntington Library, 1953), 93–114; and Herschel Baker, *The Wars of Truth* (Cambridge, Mass.: Harvard University Press, 1952), 18.

8. John Calvin, *Institutes of the Christian Religion*, trans. John Allen (Philadelphia: Presbyterian Board of Christian Education, 1936), Book 1, ch. 16, art. 2.

9. Aristotle, *Meta*. 1026b4: "We must first say regarding the *accidental*, that there can be no scientific treatment of it." See Barnes, ed., 1620–21.

10. This is the common theme of Bacon's *Novum organum*, first published in Latin in 1620. See Francis Bacon, *Novum Organum with Other Parts of the Great Instauration*, trans. Peter Urbach and John Gibson (Chicago: Open Court, 1994).

11. See Peter Dear, *Discipline and Experience* (Chicago, University of Chicago Press, 1997), 13.

12. On the importance of skepticism in the sixteenth and seventeenth centu-

ries, see Richard Popkin, *The History of Scepticism from Erasmus to Descartes,* rev. ed. (Assen: Van Gorcum, 1964).

13. A starting point for this approach has been Barbara Shapiro's *Probability and Certainty in Seventeenth-Century England* (Princeton: Princeton University Press, 1983), which identifies a concept and follows its ramifications across a variety of intellectual domains. Two other studies that I have found useful, besides the work of Daston and Park cited above, are Jean Céard's classic *La Nature et les prodiges: L'Insolite au XVIe siècle* (Genève: Librarie Droz, 1977); and Ian Hacking's *The Emergence of Probability* (New York: Cambridge University Press, 1975). As the word "genealogy" suggests, however, my approach has been influenced by the critical genealogical project proposed by Nietzsche and elaborated by Michel Foucault in his "Nietzsche, Genealogy and History." See Friedrich Nietzsche, *On the Genealogy of Morals,* trans. Walter Kaufman and R. J. Hollingdale (New York: Vintage Press, 1989), preface, section 6; and Foucault's essay in *Language, Counter-memory, Practice,* trans. Donald Bouchard and Sherry Simon (Ithaca: Cornell University Press, 1977), 139–64.

14. In the English context, we have the repeated statements of the monarch to gauge the political force of the theatrical metaphor, even if it is not directly invoked to illustrate God's providence. Elizabeth, for example, declares that "[we] princes are set on stage in the sight and view of the world," and James informs his son in his *Basilikon Doron* (1609) that kings are held up to view for the prying eyes of "spectators." (Cited in Patricia Parker, "*Othello* and *Hamlet*: Dilation, Spying, and the 'Secret Place' of Woman," *Representations* 44 [1993]: 85.)

15. The most astonishing effects seem to have been generated by objects that merged ontologically distinct categories of nature and art. This oscillation between *naturalia* and *artificialia* is described by Daston and Park in *Wonders and the Order of Nature*, ch. 7; and Joy Kenseth, "The Age of the Marvelous: An Introduction," in the *Age of the Marvelous,* 25–59, esp. 33–40. Horst Brederkamp discusses the convergence of the natural and artificial in early modern automata in his *Antikensehnsucht und Maschinenglauben: Die Geschichte der Kunstkammer und die Zukunft der Kunstgeschichte* (Berlin: Klaus Wagenbach, 1993). Paula Findlen also makes this connection with respect to objects like pieces of wood which resembled human forms in *Possessing Nature,* 95. The literary locus for the debate about the convertability of natural and artificial forms of making is Perdita's exchange with Polixines about "carnations and streaked gillyvors" in *The Winter's Tale* (4.4.79–108). See William Shakespeare, *The Complete Works,* ed. Stanley Wells and Gary Taylor (Oxford: Oxford University Press, 1988), 1118.

16. Francis Bacon, *The Advancement of Learning,* in *Francis Bacon: A Critical Edition of the Major Works,* ed. Brian Vickers (Oxford: Oxford University Press, 1996), 176.

17. The craze for curiosity collections, described in Pomian, Findlen and Park and Daston had reached England by the late sixteenth century. Walter Cope's rooms in London, for example, were filled with curiosities gathered from his travels around the world. The contents were partially described by

Thomas Platter, a resident of Basle who visited the collection in 1599. See *Thomas Platter's Travels in England, 1599*, tr. Clare Williams (London, 1937), 171–73.

18. The idea that unusual natural productions are the result of chance is mentioned in some of the materials collected by Findlen and seems to have been widespread. Bacon makes this point in the passage cited above. We see the idea that chance is a form of artistic creation put into practice, moreover, in certain paintings that merge the accidental and the deliberate, for example *Phaëthon's Fall* by Hans von Aachen, a painting on a piece of stone that incorporates natural mineral patterns as delicately unfolding clouds. The tradition of using accidental or chance patterns—for example, the spattering of paint—as a tool for artistic inspiration has a long history reaching back to Cicero's *De divinatione*, 1.13.

19. Providential hostility toward accidents is somewhat like the Victorian "repression" of sexuality described by Foucault in his *History of Sexuality:* both are an incitement to discourse. See Michel Foucault, *This History of Sexuality*, trans. Robert Hurley, vol. 1 (New York: Random House, 1978), ch. 1.

20. Jean de Chassanion, *The theatre of gods judgements: or, a collection of histories out of sacred, ecclesiasticall, and prophane authors ... Translated out of French and augmented by more than three hundred examples, by Th. Beard* (London: Adam Islip, 1597).

21. W. C., *The fatall vesper, or A true and punctuall relation of that lamentable and fearefull accident, hapning on Sunday in the afternoone being the 26. of October last, by the fall of a roome in the Black-Friers, in which were assembled many people at a sermon, which was to be preached by Father Drurie a Jesuite. Together with the names and number of such persons as therin unhappily perished, or were miraculously preserved* (London: John Haviland for Richard Whitaker, 1623), Cv–C2r.

22. John Calvin, *The institution of the Christian religion, written in Latine by M. John Calvine, and translated into English according to the authors last edition ... by Thomas Norton* (London: Arnold Hatfield: 1599), 7r.

23. For the narratological distinction, see Mieke Bal, *Narratology*, 2d ed. (Toronto: University of Toronto Press, 1997), 5, 182–87. Bal admits that it is difficult to distinguish what a narrative "event" is, but the contrast between event and action is offered as relatively conspicuous and unproblematic. I would argue that since narrative itself is often concerned with fashioning this distinction, the difference between action and event is impossible to isolate in the abstract.

24. Peter Brooks, in *Reading for the Plot: Design and Intention in Narrative* (Cambridge: Harvard University Press, 1984), makes the interesting observation that "the organizing line of plot is more often than not some scheme or machination" (12). Providentialism, as I argue in subsequent chapters, takes this structural feature of the narrative plot and asserts it as a doctrinal necessity of the world.

25. The phrase "habit of thought" is adapted from Debora Shuger's *Habits of Thought in the English Renaissance: Religion, Politics, and the Dominant Culture* (Berkeley: University of California Press, 1990). The linkage between contrivance and discovery is itself a product of the rising importance of particulars in

natural philosophy, which Daston and Park describe in *Wonders and the Order of Nature*, chs. 4 and 6.

26. Both Bacon and Gassendi were advocates of this conception of experimentation and discovery. See Eamon, *Science and the Secrets of Nature*, ch. 8. On the epistemology of this particular mode of discovery—what Carlo Ginzburg has called the "venatic method"—see his *Clues, Myths, and the Historical Method*, trans. John and Anne C. Tedeschi (Baltimore: Johns Hopkins University Press, 1989), 96–125.

27. On the dynamics of faction and intrigue in Tudor England, see Lacey Baldwin Smith, *Treason in Tudor England: Politics and Paranoia* (Princeton: Princeton University Press, 1986). On the culture of spying and its link to anxieties about infidelity, see Patricia Parker, "*Othello* and *Hamlet:* Dilation, Spying, and the 'Secret Place' of Woman." The concept of *sprezzatura* is described in Baldesar Castiglione's *Book of the Courtier* (Garden City, N.Y.: Doubleday, 1959), 43.

28. See Daston and Park, *Wonders and the Order of Nature*, ch. 8. On the classical antecedents of this belief, see Friedrich Solmsen, "Nature as Craftsman in Greek Thought," *Journal for the History of Ideas* 24, no. 4 (1963): 473–96.

29. Discourse here is used in the Foucauldian sense, referring to an area of linguistic practice that has become ordered to the point where concepts (such as that of the accident) can be regularly deployed and recognized. For a much more expansive definition of the term, see Michel Foucault, *L'Ordre du discourse* (Paris: Edition Gallimard, 1971).

30. [Thomas Goad], *The dolefull even-song, or a true particular and impartiall narration of that fearefull and sudden calamity, which befell the preacher Mr. Drury a Jesuite, and the greater part of his auditory by the downefall of the floore at an assembly in the Black-Friers on Sunday the 26 of Octob. last, in the after noone* (London: John Haviland, 1623), E2r. Arthur Freeman argues that Goad may have deliberately delayed the publication of another pamphlet and poached its details in "*The fatal vesper* and *The doleful evensong*: Claim-Jumping in 1623," *Library* 22, no. 2 (1967): 132–33.

31. Aristotle's treatment of accidental meetings in the world of deliberating beings makes his use of the metaphor immediately relevant to discussions taking place in the medieval and early modern contexts. Epicurus and Lucretius were also interested in the meeting or convergence of elements (atoms) in chance encounters, however, even if they were more widely known for the doctrine of the "swerve." See Lucretius, *De rerum natura* (2.217–24), trans. W. H. D. Rouse (Cambridge, Mass.: Harvard University Press, 1975), 112–13. In his discussion of the rediscovery of Epicurus in the sixteenth and seventeenth centuries, Jacques Lezra demonstrates how early modern Epicurianism blurred the distinction between action and event, a blurring that is characteristic of Aristotelian and Scholastic discussions of accidents as well. See Jacques Lezra, *Unspeakable Subjects: The Genealogy of the Event in Early Modern Europe* (Stanford: Stanford University Press, 1997), 1–9.

Chapter 1: Accidents and an Aristotelian Tradition

1. William Shakespeare, *Hamlet*, ed. G. R. Hibbard (New York: Oxford University Press, 1987).

2. The passage containing the line "hoist with his own petard" disappears from the Folio edition of *Hamlet;* it appears in an appendix of Hibbard's edition of the text.

3. The existential reading of this force of errancy as mere randomness, while it connects with an early modern strain of Epicurianism, sidelines the main point here: the symmetry of crime and punishment.

4. On the appetite for sudden or shocking turns of events in Elizabethan tragedy, see J. V. Cunningham, *Woe or Wonder: The Emotional Effect of Shakespearean Tragedy* (Denver: University of Denver Press, 1951), 19. I have used Patricia Parker's work on the semantic resonances of key early modern terms as a model for some of the analysis here. See, for example, her essay "*Othello* and *Hamlet:* Dilation, Spying, and the 'Secret Place' of Woman," *Representations* 44 (1993): 60–95. Parker's "resonances" tend to be synchronic—sounding across contemporary discourses and genres—whereas the ones I am charting are also understood to build up over time. This diachronic approach to semantic resonance is taken by Peggy Knapp in *Time Bound Words: Semantic and Social Economies from Chaucer's England to Shakespeare's* (New York: St. Martin's Press, 2000). Both are developing a notion introduced by Raymond Williams in his *Keywords: A Vocabulary of Culture and Society* (Oxford: Oxford University Press, 1976).

5. In identifying a learned tradition, I have grouped together different writers who focused on the logical consequences of concepts such as accident, chance, fortune, or providence. While I am uncomfortable with the elite/popular division, I conceive the learned tradition along the lines of what Peter Burke calls the "great tradition" (see Peter Burke, *Popular Culture in Early Modern Europe* [New York: New York University Press, 1978], 28), while the print sources such as pamphlets and broadsides that I treat below are understood to represent a more fluid "popular" culture of the kind described by Tessa Watt in her *Cheap Print and Popular Piety, 1550–1640* (Cambridge: Cambridge University Press, 1991), 1–3. Since I am looking at both "kinds" of text in order to trace semantic and rhetorical resonances, a number of different sources become significant and potentially comparable.

6. *The Oxford English Dictionary*, 2d ed., prepared by J. A. Simpson and E. S. C. Weiner (Oxford: Clarendon Press, 1989), 1:55. Hereafter cited as *OED*.

7. Thomas Cooper's *Thesaurus linguae Romanae & Britannicae* (London, 1565) gives a range of classical examples of the Latin *accidere* meaning "to happen," usually with the accompanying qualification "by chance," or with the sense that what happens (*accidit*) is a "misfortune."

8. It is difficult to say precisely when the generic sense of "accident" as "anything that happens" became obsolete. Since that usage was closely tied to the Aristotelian system (which differentiated the necessary from the accidental on

the basis of a metaphysical account of causation), it seems likely that the decline of this generic sense of the word is related to the decline of that system.

9. Edward Hake, *Newes out of Powles Churchyarde now newly renued and amplifyed according to the accidents of the present time. 1579. and otherwise entituled, syr Nummus. Written in English satyrs. Wherein is reprooved excessive and unlawfull seeking after riches, and the evill spending of the same. Compyled by E. H. Gent. Seene and allowed according to the order appointed* ([London]: John Charlewood and Richard Jhones, 1579); *A true report of all the proceedinges of Grave Mauris before the towne of Bercke: with all the accidentes that happened in the besiedge of the same, since the. 12. day of June last. 1601. and lastly, the yeelding up of the towne on the 30. of July following, with the conditions agreed upon betweene his excellencie and the governour of the towne. Translated out of the Dutch coppie printed at Amsterdam* (London: [R. Read?], 1601).

10. *A strange and miraculous accident happened in the cittie of Purmerent, on New-yeeres even last past 1599. Of a yong child which was heard to cry in the mothers wombe before it was borne, and about fourteene dayes of age, spake certaine sencible words, to the wonder of every body* (London: [E. Allde?], 1599).

11. Jean de Serres, *An historical collection, of the most memorable accidents, and tragicall massacres of France, under the raignes of Henry. 2. Francis. 2. Charles. 9. Henry. 3. Henry. 4. now living. Conteining all the troubles therein happened, during the said kings times, untill this present yeare, 1598. Wherein we may behold the wonderfull and straunge alterations of our age. Translated out of French into English* (London: Thomas Creede, 1598); Henry Timberlake, *A true and strange discourse of the travailes of two English pilgrimes: what admirable accidents befell them in their journey to Jerusalem, Gaza, Grand Cayro, Alexandria, and other places: also what rare antiquities, monuments, and notable memories (concording with the ancient remembrances in the holy Scriptures), they saw in Terra Sancta, with a perfect description of the old and new Jerusalem, and scituation of the countries about them. A discourse of no lesse admiration; then well worth the regarding: written by one of them, on the behalfe of himselfe, and his fellowe pilgrime* (London: [R. Bradock], 1603).

12. *Lamentable newes out of Monmouthshire in Wales. Contayning, the wonderfull and most fearefull accidents of the great overflowing of waters in the saide countye, drowning infinite numbers of cattell of all kinds, as sheepe, oxen, kine and horses, with others: together with the losse of many men, women and children, and the subversion of xxvi parishes in January last 1607* (London: [Edward Allde], 1607).

13. *More strange newes: of wonderfull accidents hapning by the late overflowings of waters, in Summerset-shire, Gloucestershire, Norfolke, and other places of England: with a true relation of the townes names that are lost, and the number of persons drowned, with other reports of accidents that were not before discovered: happening about Bristow and Barstable* (London: W[illiam] J[aggard], 1607).

14. *Newes from Italy. Or, a prodigious and most lamentable accident lately befallen: concerning the swallowing up of the whole citty of Pleurs, belonging unto the Signiory of Venice, which happened in the beginning of September last: by a strange and hidious shaking and opening of the earth. Together with the losse of more then two*

thousand people, and a generall burning up of the trees and forrests within the territories of the sayd citty. Faithfully translated out of the French copy printed at Paris. 1618 (London: N. O[kes], 1618).

15. *Newes from France. A true relation of the great losses which happened by the lamentable accident of fire in the citie of Paris, the 24. day of October last past, 1621. which burnt downe the Merchants Bridge, the Changers Bridge, and divers houses neere unto them. Together with the speedy diligence used by the Duke De Monbason, governour of the said towne, for the quenching thereof. Also a decree made in the Court of Parliament in Paris, whereby an order is taken for providing for the merchants that haue lost their goods by the sayd fire, and to prevent the like mischance in time to come. Translated according to the French copie, printed at Paris* (London: [G. Purslowe], 1621).

16. *A warning for all murderers. A most rare, strange, and wonderful accident, which by Gods just judgement was brought to passe, not farre from Rithin in Wales, and showne upon three most wicked persons, who had secretly and cunningly murdered a young gentleman named David Williams, that by no meanes it could be knowne, and how in the end it was revenged by a childe of five yeeres old, which was in his mothers wombe, and unborne when the deed was done. To the tune of, Wigmores Galliard* (London, 1620).

17. Perkins, perhaps the most influential Puritan theologian of the early seventeenth century, employed this phrase in his *A golden chaine: or, The description of theologie, containing the order of the causes of salvation and damnation, according to Gods word. A view whereof is to be seene in the table annexted. Hereunto is adjoyned the order which M. Theodore Beza sed in comforting afflicted consciences* (Cambridge: John Legat, 1600). See p. 243: "For things which in regard of men are casuall, are certainely knowne and determined by God. *Meere chaunce* is, when things are said or thought to come to passe without any cause at all. But that must be abhorred of us as overturning the providence of God." Another Puritan theologian, William Ames, advocates calling accidents contingencies in order to disentangle them from the pagan concept of fortune: "We call it a contingency so that we may avoid the error of those who commonly understand a lot to be an efficient cause which works by luck [*fortuna*]." See William Ames, *The Marrow of Theology*, trans. John D. Eusden (Durham, N.C.: Labywrinth Press, 1968), 271.

18. Or "an astrologically significant event in an individual's life." See Ann Geneva, *Astrology and the Seventeenth Century Mind* (New York: Manchester University Press, 1995), 247.

19. Giovanni Antonio Magini, *A strange and wonderfull prognostication: or rather, prenomination of those accidents which shall, or at least are likely to happen, as may be conjectured by the rules and directions of astrology, in this yeare 1624. Written by Anthonio Magini, an Italian professor of the mathematickes, and much experienced in ast[r]onomy. And now faithfully translated into English* (London: [E. Allde?], 1624).

20. Thomas Thayre, *An excellent and best approoved treatise of the plague. Containing, the nature, signes, and accidents of the same. With the certaine and absolute*

cure of the fevers, botches, and carbuncles, that raigne in these times; and above all things, most singular experiments in the same: gathered by the observations of divers worthy travilers, and selected out of the best learned physitions in this age ... (London: [N. Okes], 1625).

21. *OED*, 1:55.

22. See William Shakespeare, *The Complete Works*, ed. Stanley Wells and Gary Taylor (Oxford: Oxford University Press, 1988), 292.

23. Albert Urbanas has explored this aspect of Aristotelian logic and metaphysics extensively. See Alban Urbanas, *La Notion d'accident chez Aristote: Logique et métaphysique* (Paris: Belles Lettres, 1988).

24. On the cultural significance of these conflicts over the doctrine of "real presence," see "The Mousetrap," in Catherine Gallagher and Stephen Greenblatt, *Practicing New Historicism* (Chicago: University of Chicago Press, 2000). Early modern debates about accidental events broached some of the same questions of "signification" that Gallagher and Greenblatt raise in their essay, even if the cultural and philosophical logic governing the interpretation of temporal "accidents" was different.

25. Keith Thomas writes that after dispensing with the "apparatus of supernatural assistance" that it associated with the Catholic Church, English Protestantism had to provide its own remedies for lingering spiritual questions; the Calvinist doctrine of special providence is one such belief. (See Keith Thomas, *Religion and the Decline of Magic* [New York: Oxford University Press, 1971], 77.) On Protestant hostility to miracles, see Lorraine Daston, "Marvelous Facts and Miraculous Evidence in Early Modern Europe," *Critical Inquiry* 18, no. 1 (1991): 114–15; and Thomas, ch. 3. See also Martin Luther, *Works*, ed. Jaroslav Pelikan, vol. 21 (St. Louis: Concordia Publishing House, 1956), 280.

26. Thomas Gataker, *Of the nature and use of lots: a treatise historicall and theologicall; written by Thomas Gataker B. of D. sometime preacher at Lincolnes Inne, and now pastor of Rotherhith. The second edition* (London: John Haviland, 1627), 30–31.

27. Chapter 6 treats the accidental explanation of wonders and marvels in the early modern period at length. The idea of an "epistemic thing" is discussed by Hans-Jörg Rheinberger in his work on protein synthesis. See Hans-Jörg Rheinberger, *Toward a History of Epistemic Things: Synthesizing Proteins in the Test Tube* (Stanford: Stanford University Press, 1997). Although Rheinberger's account of experiment and experimentation would not translate directly into early modern terms, his use of the term "thing" has interesting early modern overtones.

28. We get a sense of the vastness of this flux of bodies from coney-catching manuals. Robert Greene, for example, writes in *A notable discovery of cozenage* (1591) that coney-catchers frequent St. Paul's, Fleet Street, Holborn and the Strand, where they can easily find their prey (usually a "countryman") wandering about. See Arthur Kinney, ed., *Rogues, Vagabonds, and Sturdy Beggars: A New Gallery of Tudor and Early Stuart Rogue Literature* (Amherst: University of Massachusetts Press, 1990), 167.

29. Thomas, ch. 1, esp. 15–16. Thomas paints a picture of a city rife with terrors of plague, fire and poverty. The accident literature analyzed in Chapters 4 and 6 testifies to the "theatrical" nature of many civic disasters in the early part of the seventeenth century.

30. Michael Nerlich describes the early modern boom of mercantile "adventuring" in his *Ideology of Adventure: Studies in Modern Consciousness, 1100–1750*, vol. 1, trans. Ruth Crowley (Minneapolis: University of Minnesota Press, 1987), 132–34.

31. See Aby Warburg, *The Renewal of Pagan Antiquity*, trans. David Britt (Los Angeles: Getty Research Institute, 1999), 451–65; Howard Patch, *The Goddess Fortuna in Mediaeval Literature* (Cambridge, Mass.: Harvard University Press, 1927); Samuel C. Chew, "Time and Fortune," *ELH* 6, no. 2 (1939): 83–113; Rudolf Wittkower, "Chance, Time and Virtue," *Journal of the Warburg Institute* 1 (1937–38): 313–21; Jerold C. Frakes, *The Fate of Fortune in the Early Middle Ages: The Boethian Tradition* (New York: E. J. Brill, 1988); Walter Haug, "O Fortuna," in *Fortuna*, ed. Walter Haug and Burghart Wachinger (Tübingen: Max Niemeyer Verlag, 1995), 1–22; Klaus Reichert, *Fortuna oder die Beständigkeit des Wechsels* (Frankfurt: Suhrkamp, 1985).

32. See Hanna Fenichel Pitkin, *Fortune Is a Woman: Gender and Politics in the Thought of Niccolo Machiavelli* (Chicago: University of Chicago Press, 1999), ch. 6.

33. See Joachim Theisen, "Fortuna als narratives Problem," in *Fortuna*, 143–91, for an analysis of the narratological function of Fortune in literary texts.

34. Angus Fletcher argues that allegorical agents are quasi-mechanical in his *Allegory: The Theory of a Symbolic Mode* (Ithaca: Cornell University Press, 1964), 55–57. The obvious exception to my argument that Fortune is a placeholder for absent fictional causes is the use of Fortune in philosophical dialogue, for example, in Boethius' *Consolation of Philosophy*.

35. See Niccolo Machiavelli, *The Prince*, ed. Quentin Skinner and Russell Price (Cambridge: Cambridge University Press, 1995), 87: "[F]ortune is a woman, and if you want to control her, it is necessary to treat her roughly."

36. Aby Warburg argues that the iconography of Fortune captures both the Renaissance urge for vitality and self-assertion and the medieval posture of fatalism. See Aby Warburg, 249. More recently, the idea that Fortune might be imitated (in the work of Machiavelli) has been proposed by Arlene W. Saxonhouse in her "Review of *Fortune is a Woman*, by Hanna Fenichel Pitkin," *Ethics* 105 (1985): 759–61, and in her *Women in the History of Political Thought: Ancient Greece to Machiavelli* (New York: Praeger, 1985), ch. 7.

37. See Philip Sidney, *The Old Arcadia*, ed. Katherine Duncan-Jones (New York: Oxford University Press, 1994), 10; and Maurice Evans, ed., *The Countess of Pembroke's Arcadia* (New York: Penguin Books, 1977), 61–68.

38. Such accidents happen so that the story can advance, an odd form of self-reflexive necessity that is most clearly felt in the romance's emplotment of the accident. Such a necessity is really the necessity of continuing a story: it is ultimately tied to the situation in which that story is produced or recounted.

39. The meeting takes place in Book III, Canto 7. See *Edmund Spenser's Poetry*, ed. Hugh Maclean (New York: W. W. Norton, 1968), 283.

40. Cicero, *De inventione, De optimo genere oratorum, Topica*, trans. H. M. Hubbell (Cambridge, Mass.: Harvard University Press, 1976), 30–31; [Cicero], *Ad. C. Herennium (Rhetorica ad Herennium)*, trans. Harry Caplan (Cambridge, Mass.: Harvard University Press, 1989), 44–45. The *Ad Herennium* uses *fortuna* instead of *casus*.

41. Peter Ramus, *The Logike of the Moste Excellent Philosopher P. Ramus, Martyr*, ed. Catherine M. Dunn (Northridge, Calif.: San Fernando Valley State College, 1969), 16.

42. From the twelfth to the sixteenth centuries, English homicide law recognized three kinds of homicide: culpable and therefore capital; excusable and thereby pardonable (includes killings by the insane, in self-defense, and unintentional killing); and justifiable and therefore deserving acquittal (for example, killing a known felon). Accidental killing was of the second kind and was at times pardoned "of course" or automatically upon such a finding by the jury. See Thomas Andrew Green, *Verdict According to Conscience: Perspectives on the English Criminal Trial Jury 1200–1800* (Chicago: University of Chicago Press, 1985), 86–123.

43. Green's account suggests that, although accidental or unintentional acts were recognized under the law, it was not always obvious to judges or juries what constituted an accident. This flexibility allowed juries to wrest powers from the bench in the fourteenth century, designating offenses that were clearly against the law but in their own minds justifiable "accidents" and in effect pardoning them. Aristotle discusses cases of involuntary or compulsory action, including several examples involving weapons, in *Nicomachean Ethics*, 1111a.1–21. See Barnes, ed., vol. 2, 1754.

44. See Francis Bowes Sayre, "Mens Rea," *Harvard Law Review* 45, no. 6 (1932): 974–1026.

45. Green, 88.

46. See Luke Wilson, "*Hamlet*, Hales v. Petit, and the Hysteresis of Action," *ELH* 60 (1993): 17–55.

47. I am adopting David Ross's description of Aristotle's views: "[C]hance is simply a name for the unforeseen meeting of two chains of rigorous causation." See David Ross, *Aristotle* (New York: Routledge, 1995), 80.

48. *Meta.* 1025a26–29. Aristotle, *The Complete Works of Aristotle*, ed. Jonathan Barnes (Princeton: Princeton University Press, 1984), vol. 2, 1619.

49. *Meta.* 1026b13; *Meta.* 1026b4. Barnes, ed., vol. 2, 1620–21.

50. *Phys.* 196b24–27. Barnes, ed., vol. 1, 335–36.

51. The analogy between substance and cause can be taken further, since, just as musicality might happen to be an attribute of the builder, certain events might simply happen to take place in what the builder has made. The latter are accidents of the effect, the former accidents of the cause.

52. Susan Suavé Meyer, "Aristotle, Teleology, and Reduction," *Philosophical Review* 101, no. 4 (1992): 796.

53. These two latter causes, *tuche* and *automaton*, are to be understood as species of accidental efficient causes generally conceived.

54. In a world of only one substance—for example, Spinoza's—accidents would be impossible since there would be no logically distinct causal agents to combine. There may also be accidental meetings of causal chains that do not serve any apparent purpose, although Aristotle concentrates primarily on those that do.

55. Aristotle seems to adopt a broad conception of accidental events as simply those which result when two independent lines of causality meet, as Mary Junkersfeld has argued. See M. Julienne Junkersfeld, *The Aristotelian-Thomistic Concept of Chance* (Ann Arbor, Mich.: Edwards Brothers, 1945), 76. He would probably have added, however, that such events are rare. See the example from *Meta.* 1025a14, below.

56. *Phys.* 196b33–36. Barnes, ed., vol. 1, 336. This example responds to a similar one given at the beginning of the discussion. See next footnote.

57. *Phys.* 196a2–4. Barnes, ed., vol. 1, 334. This is the example P. H. Wicksteed and F. M. Cornford believe is taken from popular comedy. See *Physics*, trans. P. H. Wicksteed and F. M. Cornford (New York: G. P. Putnam and Sons, 1929), 143.

58. *Meta.* 1025a14–17. Barnes, ed., vol. 2, 1619.

59. *Phys.* 199b19–24. Barnes, ed., vol. 1, 341.

60. Suavé Meyer, 804.

61. Medieval and early modern philosophers were interested in using possible worlds to test the logical status—the "may be" or "must be"—of certain propositions. (See Amos Funkenstein, *Theology and the Scientific Imagination* [Princeton: Princeton University Press, 1986], III.b.4–5.) Thinking in terms of possible worlds, we could say that an accident is an event that "must be" in only one possible world, but "may be" in several. The technique could be extended to provide a rhetorical theory of contingency: circumstantial descriptions of accidents specify or "pick out" the world in which accidents are necessary with respect to a particular set of circumstances. When compared with circumstances obtaining in other possible worlds, however, the accident remains a mere logical possibility.

62. *Meta.* 1027a2–5. Barnes, ed., vol. 2, 1621. Cf. Plato's example of rhetoric in the *Gorgias*, where the orator is compared to the baker, or the moment in Gorgias' *Helen* where he describes speech as a kind of magic or incantation that simply pleases its hearers and so makes them prey to fortune. (See Plato, *Gorgias*, trans. Walter Hamilton [New York: Penguin Books, 1960], 43–44; *Helen* in Patricia P. Matsen, Philip Rollinson and Marion Sousa, eds., *Readings from Classical Rhetoric* [Carbondale and Edwardsville: Southern Illinois University Press, 1990], 35). Aristotle's example is of a piece with past attempts to describe practices that produce only accidentally the good effects that a more reasoned art would bring about of necessity. Aristotle is not as pessimistic as Plato, of course, about the way in which rhetoric produces its results.

63. *Phys.* 197a24. Barnes, ed., vol. 1, 336.

64. *Meta.* 1027b4–6. Barnes, ed., vol. 2, 1622.

65. This example and the notion of an infinite temporal chain of causes that it implies will be taken up in subsequent discussions of accidents by Aquinas. Here as elsewhere, Aristotle argues ad hominem to dissolve a false infinity with the end result that an important category of events—the contingent—is saved.

66. Aristotle's use of the two terms is sometimes uneven, but most commentators agree that Aristotle held to the distinction between *tuche* and *automaton*, occasionally using *automaton* as the generic term for all events brought about by accident.

67. *Phys.* 197b16–17. Barnes, ed., vol. 1, 337.

68. Ibid., 197b14–15. The idea that animals are not capable of what Aristotle calls deliberation seems preposterous to me. The problem is taken up in the early modern period by Descartes, with similar conclusions. On the ideological significance of the animal/human divide in early modern England, see Erica Fudge, *Perceiving Animals: Humans and Beasts in Early Modern English Culture* (New York: St. Martin's Press, 2000).

69. *Phys.* 197b29–33. Barnes, ed., vol. 1, 337–38.

70. The idea that nature does so "unconsciously" is Ross's (79). There is debate about whether or not Aristotle's discussion of things "contrary to nature" in the *Physics* refers to natural anomalies like monsters. Several commentators including Philoponus, Simplicius, Albert and Aquinas assume that it does.

71. *Phys.* 197b32–36. Barnes, ed., vol. 1, 338. The argument may reflect Aristotle's practice of treating a problem with reference to the common use of terms or accepted opinions, the point here being that because *tuche* is never used to describe what is contrary to nature, the common use of the terms must reflect a difference between these two kinds of events that Aristotle himself would like to describe.

72. This hesitation at calling an internal cause a chance one appears in Hamelin, who says that monsters cannot be pure chance (*hasard*) because they have an internal efficient and final cause appropriate to their nature (Junkersfeld, 17).

73. Junkersfeld summarizes debate on this point, 17–21.

74. One warrant for including monsters under the effects of chance comes from Aristotle's *Generation of Animals*: "[T]he monstrosity, though not necessary in regard of a final cause and an end, yet is necessary accidentally." See *GA* 767b14–15. Barnes, ed., vol. 1, 1188.

75. Vincenzo Cioffari asks these questions in his *Fortune and Fate from Democritus to St. Thomas Aquinas* (New York, 1935), 17.

76. Odo Marquard makes some related remarks in his *Defense of the Accidental*: "A story is a choice that is interrupted by something accidental, something fatefully accidental; this is why stories cannot be planned, but must be told." See Odo Marquard, *In Defense of the Accidental*, trans. Robert M. Wallace (New York: Oxford University Press, 1991), 120.

77. Both accidental and intrinsic causes can fail to be hindered by certain kinds of attendant circumstances: the phase of the moon may not hinder the in-

trinsic causes of rain just as eye color might not hinder the accidental meeting. We would have to know that the accidental event was going to happen, however, before we could begin discounting certain kinds of circumstances (eye color) in advance, and this is precisely what is not possible with an accident but is possible when an intrinsic, overdetermining cause is involved.

78. *Poet.* 1452a1–10. Barnes, ed., vol. 2, 2323.

79. This metaphysics may include the idea that an author is in control of a particular fiction, but it needn't. Only in cases where the author assumes a God-like status is the metaphysics of fiction also a theology.

80. Philip Sidney, *An Apology for Poetry* (Indianapolis: Bobbs-Merrill, 1970), 32–33.

Chapter 2: Accidents from Cicero to Calvin

1. *Institutes*, Book I, ch. 17, art. 10. See John Calvin, *Institutes of the Christian Religion*, trans. John Allen, vol. 1 (Philadelphia: Presbyterian Board of Christian Education, 1936), 245.

2. Calvin's considerable knowledge of the Scholastic tradition is described in William J. Bouwsma, *John Calvin: A Sixteenth Century Portrait* (New York: Oxford University Press, 1988), 101–2. Calvin's debt to Augustine in the *Institutes* is obvious; he glosses Augustine's analysis of chance and fortune, for example, in *Institutes*, Book I, ch. 16, art. 8. Allen, trans., 228.

3. Calvin is not the only Reformation theologian to take an interest in providence. On the centrality of providence in the writings of Protestant historians (Foxe, Melanchthon, Sleidan, Crespin), see A. G. Dickens, John Tonkin, with Kenneth Powell, *The Reformation in Historical Thought* (Cambridge: Harvard University Press, 1985), 47. Luther's interest in the actuality (rather than the potentiality) of providence is discussed in Paul Althaus, *The Theology of Martin Luther*, trans. Robert C. Shultz (Philadelphia: Fortress Press, 1966), 110–11.

4. See Peggy Knapp, *Time Bound Words: Semantic and Social Economies from Chaucer's England to Shakespeare's* (New York: St. Martin's Press, 2000), 118–19. The phrase "mode of civic consciousness" belongs to J. G. A. Pocock, quoted in Knapp, 118.

5. Perhaps the best documented case is that of Nehemiah Wallington, a seventeenth-century Puritan artisan who kept extensive diaries chronicling his encounters with providence. See Paul Seaver, *Wallington's World: A Puritan Artisan in Seventeenth-Century London* (Stanford: Stanford University Press, 1985), ch. 3. While Wallington's is an extreme case, the providential sensibility he expresses is not. On the prevalence of providentialism outside of Puritan circles, see Lotte Mulligan, "Puritans and English Science: A Critique of Webster," *ISIS* 71, no. 258 (1980): 456–69, esp. 462–65.

6. The details surrounding such accidents might undergo minor changes in subsequent discussion, for example when Albert writes that it is Demosthenes and Eschinus who meet in the forum rather than two unnamed "someones." The practice of textual commentary, however, serves a fundamentally conser-

vational purpose: it ensures that these canonical examples are retained and quibbled with instead of being abandoned or spontaneously revised.

7. At least six English writers, including Elizabeth herself, produced translations of this book between 1525 and 1609. The first such edition to appear was a translation by J. Walton in 1525; next follows an edition by George Colville in 1556, of which a second edition followed five years later. Subsequent editions, besides the translation by Elizabeth, include Sir Thomas Chaloner's (1563), Bracegirdle's (1604) and that of I. T. (1609), which I quote here. Geoffrey Chaucer also produced a translation that was published by Caxton in 1478: very little of the Latinate technical vocabulary surrounding accidents appears in his explanation of the accident. For example, a key passage from Book V quoted below is translated by Chaucer as the "causes of the abbreging of foruyn happe," which the sixteenth-century writer translates as the "causes" of the "fortunate accident." See Boethius, *Boecius de consolacione philosophie* ([Westminster: William Caxton], 1478), K6r.

8. Anicius Manlius Severinus Boethius, *The Consolation of Philosophy*, ed. William Anderson, trans. I. T. (Carbondale, Ill.: Southern Illinois University Press, 1963), 105–6. The Latin is from Anicii Manlii Severnini Boethii, *Philosophiae consolatio*, ed. Ludovicus Bieler (Turnholti: Typographi Brepols Editores Pontificii, 1957), 89.

9. Jerold Frakes points out that the specific phrase, *ex confluentibus causis*, belongs to Aristotle's commentators. See Jerold C. Frakes, *The Fate of Fortune in the Early Middle Ages: The Boethian Tradition* (New York: E. J. Brill, 1998), 59.

10. Anderson, ed., 106.

11. Paradoxically, Fate in Boethius' story becomes an arrangement of movable things, a necessity of one's place and time that one really possesses—one cannot presumably be somewhere else, or in another time—but that is not a consequence of one's nature or will. On the Stoic conception of providence, see the corresponding chapter in A. A. Long, *Hellenistic Philosophy: Stoics, Epicureans, Sceptics* (New York: Charles Scribner's Sons, 1974).

12. Allen, trans., 220.

13. Creation, Calvin writes, "belongs no less to [God's] hands than to his eyes." Allen, trans., 222.

14. Ibid., 232.

15. This process of appropriating "paradigmatic" examples of the nature of experience is elegantly described in Hans Blumenberg's *Shipwreck with Spectator: Paradigm of a Metaphor for Existence* (Cambridge: MIT Press, 1997).

16. See Eleonor Stump's Introduction to Boethius, *Boethius's In Ciceronis Topica*, trans. Eleonore Stump (Ithaca: Cornell University Press, 1988), 6–7.

17. When pleading a case, one has often to distinguish between two kinds of efficient causes: those that are sufficient to bring about an effect, and others such as chance and fortune that are merely necessary. See Cicero, *De inventione, De optimo genere oratorum, Topica*, trans. H. M. Hubbell (Cambridge, Mass.: Harvard University Press, 1976), 424–27. Subsequent references to this text appear parenthetically in the text.

18. Cicero gives a variety of examples of particularly credible evidence that is given of "necessity" or inadvertently, for example when children give important information without knowing its pertinence, when one makes incriminating statements while someone else is listening through a wall, or when one talks while drunk or in one's sleep (Hubbell, trans., 438–41). On inartificial or nontechnical modes of persuasion, see Aristotle, *The Rhetoric and Poetics of Aristotle*, trans. W. Rhys Roberts and Ingram Bywater (New York: McGraw Hill, 1984), 24. On inartificial proofs in the context of Renaissance dialectic, see R. W. Serjeantson, "Testimony and Proof in Early-Modern England," *Studies in History and Philosophy of Science* 30, no. 2 (1999): 195–236, esp. 203.

19. Joel Altman has written about the relationship between improvisation in the play and the process of its composition, with particular emphasis on the rhetorical concept of *kairos*. See Joel B. Altman, "'Preposterous Conclusions': Eros, *Enargeia*, and the Composition of *Othello*," *Representations* 18 (1987): 129–57. Clearly accidents are *kairotic* occasions for improvisation in the play, as well as a stimulus to narrative. I would add that they are occasions for discovery.

20. Albertus Magnus, *Physica*, ed. Paulus Hossfeld (Aschendorff: Monasterii Westfalorum, 1987), 114.

21. Even if the pilot of one of Boethius' ships has a will of his own, they might argue, he may have been born under a star that destines him for a particular meeting several leagues downstream. In addition to the necessity of the stars, Albert recognizes a *complexio causarum* that knits events together in what the Stoics call Fate. Because Fate exerts an unequal pull on objects (given the variations of matter), however, it does not eradicate accidental contingency of the kind Aristotle describes. Fate is thus nonbinding. See Vincenzo Cioffari, *Fortune and Fate from Democritus to St. Thomas Aquinas* (New York, 1935), 94.

22. Hossfeld, ed., 114. See Cioffari, 95–97, for a fuller discussion of Albert's simultaneous commitment to astrological necessity and Aristotelian chance.

23. Hossfeld, ed., 114: "Sit enim pater familias dives habens servos plurimos habeatque pecora in foveis iacentia ignorantibus servis, quae tamen vult, ut extrahant servi, quando inveniunt. Revelat autem servis ad eundem ad locum foveae, in qua iacent animalia, et non revelat eis causam, quare vadant illuc, nec revelat uni, quod alter veniat ad locum, sed divisim revelat eis ire ad locum per diversas vias. Illorum enim servorum unus alium non intendit invenire iuxta foveam, nec aliquis intendit extrahere animalia de fovia, quia nesciunt ea cecidisse in foveam. Et ideo casu extrahunter animalia de fovia quantum ad eos et salvanter, et casu se invicem inveniunt iuxta foveam, et tamen quoad patrem familias nihil horum est casu." [English translation by author]

24. *Physics*, lib. 2, tract. 2, cap. 10: Hoc autem, si verum est, tunc perit liberum arbitrium et perit consilium, sicut et perit casus et perit fortuna. Hossfeld, ed., 114.

25. *Physics*, lib. 2, tract. 2, cap. 21. In doing so Albert insists that foreseeing something does not impose necessity on it [*praescientia nullam rebus imponit necessitatem*] (129), much as Augustine does in his discussion of providence in *City of God*, Book 5, ch. 10. (See Augustine, *City of God*, trans. Henry Bettenson

[Baltimore: Penguin Classics, 1976], 195.) God's foresight works outside of time—he sees what will happen as if in an eternal present—and so from this point of view future accidents could be said to happen inexorably [*immobiliter*].

26. Thomas Aquinas, *Selected Philosophical Writings*, trans. Timothy McDermott (New York: Oxford University Press, 1993), 280.

27. Most likely, it will simply be postponed. At some point Aquinas would have to explain the relationship between God's knowledge of what will happen and his preference for the outcome that results. Aquinas's response would most likely have to be that God chooses a world in which all contingent facts are to his liking. Leibniz made this moment of divine choice the starting point for contingency in a world that God chooses because it contains the greatest number of compossibles. On the significance of this initial choice in Leibniz's theory and its relationship to his distinction between absolute and hypothetical necessity, see Amos Funkenstein, *Theology and the Scientific Imagination* (Princeton: Princeton University Press, 1986), 103, 146.

28. *Summa theologiae*, I, quest. 86, art. 4. See Thomas Aquinas, *Summa theologiae*, 60 vols., trans. and ed. Fathers of the English Dominican province (New York: McGraw-Hill, 1964), 12:99–103; hereafter cited as *ST*.

29. The classic example of an accidental unity is Socrates sitting, although there are others. For a contemporary evaluation of the problem of whether or not accidental unities ("kooky objects") are one thing, see Gareth B. Matthews, "Accidental Unities," in *Language and Logos*, ed. Malcolm Schofield and Martha Craven Nussbaum (New York: Cambridge University Press, 1982), 223–40.

30. McDermott, trans., 282.

31. The epistemological warrant for this claim is the idea that our knowledge of contingent events is immediate and sensory when those events are singular, but becomes abstract and intellectual only when there is something necessary about those events. (See *ST*, I, quest. 86, art. 3. Fathers of the English Dominican province, trans., 98–99.) Another version of the argument I am tracing here is that accidents are singulars and so can only be known by us through the senses, whereas God knows such singulars from eternity. Accidents have no abstract content and so have nothing to offer the philosopher. See, however, Amos Funkenstein's remarks about God's knowledge of singular things (rather than events) in relation to his role as *artifex* in *Theology and the Scientific Imagination*, 137.

32. As Bert Hansen comments in his critical edition of this work, Oresme was not the first to try to naturalize marvels in this manner, and he points to similar impulses in Lucretius, Seneca, Augustine, Adelard of Bath, and Roger Bacon. See Bert Hansen, *Nicole Oresme and the Marvels of Nature: A Study of His De Causis Mirabilium with Critical Edition, Translation, and Commentary* (Toronto: Pontifical Institute of Mediaeval Studies, 1985), 64–73.

33. Lorraine Daston and Katherine Park, *Wonders and the Order of Nature, 1150–1750* (New York: Zone Books, 1998), 131, hereafter cited as *WO*.

34. See Hansen, 228–29.

35. *Summa contra gentiles*, III, quest. 99, art. 9. See Thomas Aquinas, *Summa*

contra gentiles, trans. Vernon J. Bourke, vol. 3:2 (Notre Dame: University of Notre Dame Press, 1975), 78–79.

36. *Physics*, 2.1.17. Quoted in *WO*, 116.

37. See, for example, Edward Fenton's "Epistle Dedicatorie" to Pierre Boaistuau, *Certain secrete wonders of nature, containing a descriptio[n] of sundry strange things, seming monstrous in our eyes and judgement, bicause we are not privie to the reasons of them* (London: Henry Bynneman, 1569). Jean Céard discusses the ideas of both Boaistuau and Lycosthenes in *La Nature et les prodiges: L'Insolite au XVIe siècle, en France* (Genève: Librarie Droz, 1977), chs. 7, 10. On monsters as a model of cooperation, see *WO*, 192.

38. See *The Advancement of Learning*, Book II, in *Francis Bacon: A Critical Edition of the Major Works*, ed. Brian Vickers (Oxford: Oxford University Press, 1996), 176–77.

39. Martin Luther and Philipp Melanchthon, *Deuttung der czwo grewlichen figuren, Bapstesels czu Rom und Munchkalbs zu Freijberg in Meijsszen funden*, in *D. Martin Luthers Werke*, 102 vols. to date (Weimar: H. Bohlau, 1883–), vol. 1, pt. 11, 369–85. On Luther's polemical use of the deformed cow fetus, see Ottavia Niccoli, *Prophecy and People in Renaissance Italy*, trans. Lydia G. Cochrane (Princeton: Princeton University Press, 1990), 122–26.

40. See [Aristotle], *The problems of Aristotle with other philosophers and physitians: wherein are contained divers questions, with their answers, touching the estate of mans body* (London: John Raworth, 1638); and Ambroise Paré, *On Monsters and Marvels*, trans. Janis L. Pallister (Chicago: University of Chicago Press, 1982), 14–15.

41. Allen, trans., 225–26.

42. William Bouwsma situates this knowledge in the context of early modern skepticism, whereas Edward A. Dowey offers a dialectical reading of knowledge in Calvin's theology, opposing knowledge of God as creator in his works to a knowledge of him as redeemer. See William J. Bouwsma, *John Calvin: A Sixteenth Century Portrait* (New York: Oxford University Press, 1988); and Edward A. Dowey, Jr., *The Knowledge of God in Calvin's Theology* (Grand Rapids, Mich.: Wm. B. Eerdmans Publishing, 1994).

43. Bouwsma refers to this experimental knowledge that leads to faith on p. 158. Calvin distinguishes between knowledge of faith [*scientia fidei*] and experimental knowledge [*scientia experimentalis*] in *Comm. Zech.* 2:9. See vol. 72 of *Corpus reformatorum*, ed. Baum et al., 87 vols. (Brunsvigae: C. A. Schwetschke et filium, 1863–1900), 162.

44. Allen, trans., 230.

45. "For the Lord is manifested by his perfections: perceiving the influence and enjoying the benefits of which, we must necessarily be more acutely impressed with such a knowledge, than if we imagined a Deity of whose influence we had no perception." Allen, trans., 72.

46. Stump, trans., 163; See also *ST*, I, quest. 115, art. 6; Fathers of the English Dominican province, trans., vol. 15, 114–15.

47. The nature of this kind of knowledge is not simply intellectual—the seat of this knowledge is the heart—but clearly Calvin intends such a *scientia* to be as much a cognitive conviction as it is a feeling of being persuaded or affected by God's presence. See Bouwsma, ch. 9.

48. *Inst.* Book I, ch. 5, art. 8. Allen, trans., 71. The French is from Jean Calvin, *Institution de la religion Chretienne, livre premier*, ed. Jean-Daniel Benoit (Paris: Librarie Philosophique J. Vrin, 1957), 76; the Latin from Jean Calvin, *Institutio Christianae religionis in libros quatuor*, vol. 30, *Corpus reformatorum*, 47.

49. Allen, trans., 72. Elsewhere he will quote Augustine extensively concerning the secret order of chance or fortune—"concurrences ordained." Allen, trans., 228–29.

50. Allen, trans., 368.

51. Bouwsma, 172.

Chapter 3: The Avoidance of Ends

1. *Gesta Grayorum* (1688), v–vi, excerpted in R. A. Foakes, ed., *The Comedy of Errors* (Cambridge, Mass.: Harvard University Press, 1940), 116. All quotations from *The Comedy of Errors* are taken from William Shakespeare, *The Complete Works*, ed. Stanley Wells and Gary Taylor (Oxford: Clarendon Press, 1988). Quotations from other plays by Shakespeare are found in this edition.

2. Harold Jenkins, "Shakespeare's *Twelfth Night*," in *Shakespeare: The Comedies: A Collection of Critical Essays*, ed. Kenneth Muir (Englewood Cliffs, N.J.: Prentice Hall, 1959), 73. See also Russ McDonald, "Fear of Farce," in *"Bad" Shakespeare*, ed. Maurice Charney (London: Associated University Presses, 1988), 77–90.

3. The diagnoses of an excessive reliance on the arbitrary is reiterated by several critics. See, for example, Francis Fergusson, *The Human Image in Dramatic Literature* (Gloucester, Mass.: Peter Smith, 1969), 149: "The foolishness presented in this play is that of the incredible and arbitrary basic situation, not the ineluctable folly of mankind." See also C. L. Barber, "Shakespearian Comedy in *The Comedy of Errors*," *College English* 25, no. 7 (1964), 493, on the "arbitrary imposition" of the plot on the action of the play. Other critics have felt obliged to point out what seems to be an excessive reliance on plot. Hazlitt, for example, writes that *The Comedy of Errors* does not often demonstrate Shakespeare's "genius," since in it he "seems to have relied on his author, and on the interest arising out of the intricacy of the plot." See William Hazlitt, *Characters of Shakespeare's Plays*, 2d ed. (London: Taylor & Hessey, 1818), 260. D. J. Palmer quotes H. B. Charlton to the effect that "the plot becomes a sort of mathematical exhibition of the maximum number of erroneous combinations of four people in pairs." See D. J. Palmer, "The Early Comedies," in *Shakespeare: Select Bibliographical Guides*, ed. Stanley Wells (Oxford: Oxford University Press, 1973), 59. Finally, K. T. von Rosador is obliged to defend the play against having gone too far in the direction of mechanical plotting, outlining the "plot strategies" that the playwright employs to "counteract such mechanization." See K. Tetzeli von

Rosador, "Plotting the Early Comedies: 'The Comedy of Errors,' 'Love's Labour's Lost,' 'The Two Gentlemen of Verona,'" *Shakespeare Survey* 37 (1984): 16–17.

4. Samuel Taylor Coleridge, *Shakespearean Criticism*, 2 vols. (New York: E. P. Dutton, 1960), I:89.

5. Both early modern and contemporary theorists of comedy have maintained the importance of accident in the genre. Guarini's identification of accident, passion, fortune and the character of events themselves as the sources of comedy is quoted in Leo Salingar, *Shakespeare and the Traditions of Comedy* (Cambridge: Cambridge University Press, 1974), 87. Salingar himself believes that Shakespeare's comedies "depend at some point on chance, which is a regular leading agent alongside the characters" (20). Kenneth Muir also identifies "accidents" as a common feature of comedy, arguing that in this genre "the mutual happiness of lovers, expected by the audience at the end of the last act, may be postponed by quarrels, misunderstandings, separations, disguises, and accidents." See Kenneth Muir, "Comic Tradition and the European Context: The Testing of Love," in *Comedy from Shakespeare to Sheridan*, ed. A. R. Braunmuller and J. C. Bulman (Newark, N.J.: University of Delaware Press, 1986), 72.

6. Sylvia, when apprehended by the outlaws, says defiantly, "A thousand more mischances than this one / Have learned me how to brook this patiently" in *The Two Gentlemen of Verona* (5.3.2–3). Her patience in the face of chance here is an instance of the Renaissance opposition of virtue and patience to chance. Since it is true that the outlaws plan to ambush someone, their doing so is no accident; the fact that it is Valentine whom they manage to get hold of is an accident, however.

7. As Bertrand Evans has remarked, the plot advances in this play without a "practiser" or deceiver. See Bertrand Evans, *Shakespeare's Comedies* (Oxford: Clarendon Press, 1960), 3. This discrepancy between different levels of knowledge in the play suggests that Niklas Luhmann is right when he asserts that the problem of contingency emerges only when one is observing a process of observation. See Niklas Luhmann, *Observations on Modernity*, trans. William Whobrey (Stanford: Stanford University Press, 1998), 47. Such a discrepancy is implied in many of the Scholastic examples of accidents as well.

8. C. L. Barber recognizes the obstacle posed by understanding when he says that perpetuating the farcical confusion in this play "requires that each person involved be shown making some sort of sense out of it, while failing to see through it as an audience can" (494). Again and again characters find their expectations frustrated, and yet the confusion always bears the stamp of some deeper purpose. Adriana, for example, suspects her husband of infidelity when his twin denies that he has a wife (2.1); the Antipholuses think their bondmen are intentionally tricking them or are jesting inappropriately when orders get confused (1.2, 2.2); the Merchant thinks Antipholus of Ephesus is trying to steal from him when he is refused payment (4.1); Antipholus of Ephesus thinks his wife is entertaining "customers" when he is locked out of his house (4.4); more than one person is willing to believe that Antipholus of Ephesus is possessed by

demons when he is angered at his arrest (4.4); and Pauline lore about witchcraft in Ephesus is repeated by the Syracusans when they cannot understand the strange events they see (1.2).

9. Bacon discusses the Idols in the *Novum organum*, Book 1, Aphorisms 52–62. See Francis Bacon, *Novum Organum with Other Parts of the Great Instauration*, ed. Peter Urbach and John Gibson (Chicago: Open Court, 1994), 61–68. Bacon's "Device for the Gray's Inn Revels" appears in *Francis Bacon: A Critical Edition of the Major Works*, ed. Brian Vickers (New York: Oxford University Press, 1996), 52–60. On the spiritual resonances of error in the play, see Steven R. Shelburne, "The Nature of 'Error' in *The Comedy of Errors*," *Explorations in Renaissance Culture* 18 (1992): 137–51.

10. Ann Barton, "Introduction to *The Comedy of Errors*," in *The Riverside Shakespeare*, ed. G. Blakemore Evans (Boston: Houghton Mifflin, 1974), 79.

11. Most critics emphasize some sense of social realignment at the ending of the play. See for example W. Thomas MacCary, "*The Comedy of Errors*: A Different Kind of Comedy," *New Literary History* 9, no. 3 (1978): 525–36. Stephen Greenblatt points to the social mechanisms of this alignment in his introduction to the play in *The Norton Shakespeare*. (See William Shakespeare, *The Norton Shakespeare*, ed. Stephen Greenblatt [New York: W. W. Norton, 1997], 683–89.) See also Douglas Lanier on the play's interrogation of the material underpinnings of identity in Elizabethan England: "'Stigmatical in Making': The Material Character of *The Comedy of Errors*," *English Literary Renaissance* 23, no. 1 (1993): 81–112.

12. Gamini Salgado, "'Time's Deformed Hand': Sequence, Consequence, and Inconsequence in 'The Comedy of Errors,'" *Shakespeare Survey* 25 (1972): 82.

13. Jonathan V. Crewe, "God or the Good Physician: The Rational Playwright in *The Comedy of Errors*," *Genre* 15, no. 1/2 (1982): 213. Egeon believes that his story is so predictable or generic that he does not need to finish it. Halfway through the tale he tells the Duke, "O, let me say no more! / Gather the sequel by that went before" (1.1.94–95).

14. Following Marvin T. Herrick, Eamon Grennan notes the strict, self-conscious way in which the conventional rhetorical form is observed and embellished. See Eamon Grennan, "Arm and Sleeve: Nature and Custom in *The Comedy of Errors*," *Philological Quarterly* 59, no. 2 (1980): 156–57.

15. *OED*, first and second definitions.

16. Crewe argues that Egeon's melancholic view of a consistently punishing Fortune is at odds with the romance conventions he is invoking (213–14). In effect, there can be nothing contingent about a Fortune that acts so uniformly.

17. The haps of the narrative are, in Egeon's self-conscious presentation, the material precondition for their own representation. One might think ahead to Bacon's painting of shipwreck survivors in the *New organon*, Book I, Aphorism 46, which emphasizes just this material link between the events that befall a person and the potential for their representation in that person's survival. See Urbach et al., eds., 57–58. On the preposterous in early modern rhetoric and

Shakespearean drama, see Patricia Parker, *Literary Fat Ladies: Rhetoric, Gender, Property* (New York: Methuen, 1987), 93–96.

18. While the significance attached to Egeon's presence is preposterous, his conclusion rests on an interesting and quite reasonable assumption: explanations of past events must be compatible with the present fact that someone is around to speak about them (a rhetorical version of the weak anthropic principle). This assumption focuses our attention on another crucial area of disconnect in the play, since error surfaces repeatedly at the moment when a speaker must in fact *be* the person described at the end of a narrative of past events. Stories about the speaker must end with that speaker, but this matter-of-fact convergence of representer with represented—it is ultimately another kind of meeting of twins—gets forestalled when no one knows who that speaker really is. Audiences will see and hear this missed meeting again and again as spoken narratives "round the bend" and speakers explain how they finally came to arrive in their present situation.

19. Among other things, the play is an extended gloss on the philosophical ambiguity of the word "and" in narrative description.

20. See Patricia Parker, "Anagogic Metaphor: Breaking Down the Wall of Partition," in *Centre and Labyrinth: Essays in Honour of Northrop Frye*, ed. E. Cook et al. (Toronto: University of Toronto Press, 1983), 38–58; "Shakespeare and the Bible: *The Comedy of Errors*," *Recherches sémiotiques/Semiotic Inquiry* 13, no. 3 (1993): 47–72. On the general connection between romance and "dilation," see her *Inescapable Romance: Studies in the Poetics of a Mode* (Princeton: Princeton University Press, 1979), 8–10.

21. Dromio of Ephesus' characteristic mode of speech is *parataxis*, an affectation that suggests an ironic distance from events as they unfold. See, for example, 3.1.71: "Your cake here is warm within: you stand here in the cold" or 4.1.21: "I buy a thousand pound a year! I buy a rope!" In Renaissance rhetoric, this manner of speaking would probably have been identified as a species of *eclipsis* such as *dissolutio* (*asyndeton*). See, for example, Thomas Wilson, *The Arte of Rhetorique* (1560), ed. G. H. Mair (Oxford: Oxford University Press, 1909), 205.

22. The trope of *gradiatio* has been used in philosophical argumentation to ridicule the Stoic idea of an unbreakable causal sequence. Aquinas, for example, following Aristotle, rejects the idea that everything happens as it must by describing one of the consequences of this view: "If, for example, someone who has eaten salt will thirst, and someone thirsty will go out to get a drink, and someone going out will get killed by robbers, then, because he has already eaten the salt, he is bound to get killed." See Thomas Aquinas, *Selected Philosophical Writings*, trans. Timothy McDermott (Oxford: Oxford University Press, 1993), 279.

23. The latter fact, incidentally, has nothing to do with the presence of a twin; it is perhaps the only intentional offense that Antipholus of Ephesus gives Adriana in the play.

24. That the limit appears so clearly in this play suggests just how powerful

this mode of reasoning was becoming. Barbara Shapiro has explored the role of probable reasoning in the fields of law, rhetoric, theology and natural philosophy in her *Probability and Certainty in Seventeenth-Century England* (Princeton: Princeton University Press, 1983). The mistakes in this play mark an important blind spot in this mode of reasoning, since appeals to probability assume a mismatch between the improbable and the believable. The play demonstrates how, unsurprisingly, the improbable resists explanation by the even more improbable.

25. Once these stories get told, characters may or may not recognize themselves in them. A great deal rides on such recognitions, since in a play where social class, dress, name and the body itself fail to individuate, memories and the stories that make those memories public would be the only source of communally recognized identity.

26. When asked why he is beating Dromio of Syracuse, for example, Antipholus of Syracuse responds: "Why, first: for flouting me; and then 'wherefore': / For urging it the second time to me" (2.2.45–46). That first offense was itself one of telling an outrageous story. When Dromio of Ephesus tells Antipholus of Syracuse about his "wife," he responds, "What, wilt thou flout me thus unto my face, / Being forbid? There, take you that, sir knave" (1.2.91–93).

27. The law students at the Gray's Inn revels would probably have found this and the opposing *narratio* that follows entertaining, since their legal training involved similar exercises of "case-putting" or "moots," the latter a formal exercise in which two students or barristers argued opposing sides of a case before two or three utter-barristers or benchers sitting as judges. See Wilfred R. Prest, *The Inns of Court under Elizabeth I and the Early Stuarts: 1590–1640* (Totawa, N.J.: Rowman and Littlefield, 1972), 117. The cause that she pleads covers a mix of Ciceronian judicial topics that would have been well known to some of the students. In that she wants to establish that Antipholus has done certain things and that the Abbess has done others, she is concerned with an issue of fact (*constitutio conjecturalis*). However, by admitting certain facts but qualifying them, showing that Antipholus is acting dangerously because he is mad, she is also concerned with the nature and quality of the act (*constitutio generalis*). Finally, Adriana's attempts to persuade the Duke that it is his responsibility to remedy the situation might be seen as an issue of translation (*constitutio translativa*), since it pertains to the propriety of time or venue for a given plea. See Cicero, *De inventione,* trans. H. M. Hubbell (Cambridge: Harvard University Press, 1976), 20–23. All three issues are taken up in the twenty-four-line *narratio* that briefly, as Cicero recommends, relates the sequence of events in the order that they occurred (54–63). Cicero, in discussing what not to do in a judicial *narratio,* gives a rambling version of an exchange between a man inquiring of a slave if his master is home (59), the same incident that creates discord in this play.

28. That he makes provisional sense of the confusion by referring to another story is itself worth noting.

29. This is Derrida's point in "Signature, Event, Context," one that he claims

is implicit in Austin's *How to Do Things With Words*. Derrida's essay appears in *Limited Inc* (Evanston, Ill.: Northwestern University Press, 1990). See in particular his argument that Austin's account of performatives excludes the risk of infelicity as merely "accidental" or contextual rather than a structural possibility (14–15).

30. While Antipholus may be wrong in his suspicions, he is nonetheless telling a true story about what happened to him. Joel Altman has remarked how both sides in the legal pleading are telling the truth. See Joel Altman, *The Tudor Play of Mind* (Berkeley: University of California Press, 1978), 171.

31. Cicero argues that the fact of a criminal act may be admitted and yet punishment withheld if the act can be shown to have been done in ignorance, by accident (*casum*) or out of necessity. In his elaborate hierarchy of judicial issues, Cicero places this plea from "imprudentiam, casum, necessitatem" in the category of *purgatio*, a kind of *concessio* that belongs to the assumptive portion of equitable pleas. See Hubbell, trans., 30–31. The pseudo-Ciceronian *Rhetorica ad Herennium* recognizes *casus* as a legitimate legal topic as well. See [Cicero], *De ratione dicendi* (*Rhetorica ad Herennium*), trans. Harry Caplan (Cambridge: Harvard University Press, 1989), 44–45.

32. For an analysis of the importance of *kairos* in ancient rhetorical theory, see Mario Untersteiner, *The Sophists*, trans. Kathleen Freeman (Oxford: Basil Blackwell, 1954), 111–12, 118–21, 177–78. A synoptic treatment emphasizing the importance of *kairos* within contemporary rhetorical theory, pedagogy and literary criticism appears in James L. Kinneavy's "*Kairos*: A Neglected Concept in Classical Rhetoric," in *Rhetoric and Praxis: The Contribution of Classical Rhetoric to Practical Reasoning*, ed. Jean Dietz Moss (Washington: Catholic University of America Press, 1986), 79–105.

33. The traditional narratological distinction between the sequence of events and the sequence of their presentation—what is known as plot—depends precisely on this indifference of narrative sequence to the kind of "extra-discursive necessity" that governs the sequence of events described.

Chapter 4: *Hamlet* Interrupted

1. Unless otherwise noted, references to *Hamlet* are to the following edition: *Hamlet*, ed. G. R. Hibbard (New York: Oxford University Press, 1987). Hibbard's text excludes Q2 passages cut from the Folio, so my arguments should be construed as applying to F.

2. Most critics are faced with the choice of interpreting conscience as meaning either "consciousness" or as the faculty of moral judgment. I do not favor excluding the first definition, since it resonates with the sense of "regard" as consciously attending to something. The extraordinary range of meanings for the word "regard" in this period cited in the *OED* (8:364–65)—meaning to look at, notice, value, have care for, take heed of, or contemplate with feeling—is being exploited with great subtlety when "regard" is placed in a parallel construction with "conscience." For a critique of the reading I am choosing, see

Catherine Belsey, "The Case of Hamlet's Conscience," *Studies in Philology* 76, no. 2 (1979): 127–48.

3. I have chosen the word "distraction" here partly in deference to early modern usage, where the term indicated a "pulling apart." It is tempting to describe this attendant awareness of artifice in theatrical consciousness in terms of belief and disavowal, as is sometimes done in psychoanalytic film theory. Christian Metz, for example, has argued that the cinematic spectator experiences a divided belief in the images that are projected on screen. On one level, he or she knows that what is represented is not real—that it lacks reality. But on another level, he or she is still credulous and so can be said to disavow that lack. (See Christian Metz, *The Imaginary Signifier: Psychoanalysis and the Cinema*, trans. Celia Britton, Annwyl Williams, Ben Brewster, and Alfred Guzzetti [Bloomington: University of Indiana Press, 1982], 71–72.) As Metz himself suggests, however, it is more difficult to effect such a disavowal in the theater because of the physical presence of "real" actors. It thus seems more appropriate to describe theatrical consciousness not in terms of levels of knowledge or disavowal but as a phenomenological tug of war in which the physical conditions of performance (actors, stage, audience) and extratheatrical concerns (historical, religious, political) make simultaneous and competing claims on consciousness. My own use of "distraction" as a theoretical term should not be understood as a forerunner of modern "distraction" as analyzed by Walter Benjamin and others. I do, however, see this analysis as part of a larger history of attention and the cultural practices associated with its manipulation. On the latter, see Jonathan Crary, *Suspensions of Perception: Attention, Spectacle, and Modern Culture* (Boston: MIT Press, 1999).

4. "Hamlet's capture by the pirates. This is almost the only play of Shakespeare, in which mere accidents, independent of all will, form an essential part of the plot." See S. T. Coleridge, *Notes and Lectures upon Shakespeare*, ed. H. N. Coleridge, vol. 2 (London: William Pickering, 1849), 235.

5. A. C. Bradley, *Shakespearean Tragedy* (London: Macmillan, 1985), 140: "[It] appears probable that the 'accident' is meant to impress the imagination as the very reverse of the accidental, and with many readers it certainly does so. And that this was the intention is made the more likely by a second fact, the fact that in connection with the events of the voyage Shakespeare introduces that feeling, on Hamlet's part, of his being in the hands of Providence."

6. The readings of this moment differ in emphasis, some critics remarking the surrender to providence, others emphasizing an openness to chance or a discovery of the power of the will, while still others emphasize Hamlet's Stoic resolve. The surrender to providence is most completely argued in Bertram Joseph, *Conscience and the King* (London: Chatto and Windus, 1953), 130–51. Critics emphasizing accident, chance or indeterminacy are Strachey (quoted in Furness's gloss on these lines; see *Hamlet*, ed. Horace Howard Furness, vol. 2, *A New Variorum Edition of Shakespeare* [Philadelphia: J. B. Lippincott, 1918], 172–74); John Hunt, "A Thing of Nothing: The Catastrophic Body in *Hamlet*," *Shake-*

speare Quarterly 39, no. 1 (1988): 42; and William Beatty Warner, *Chance and the Text of Experience: Freud, Nietzsche, and Shakespeare's Hamlet* (Ithaca: Cornell University Press, 1986), 268–75. Arguments about Hamlet's greater confidence in the will are to be found in Richard Mallette, "From Gyves to Graces: *Hamlet* and Free Will," *Journal of English and Germanic Philology* 93, no. 3 (1994): 336–55. The Stoic sense appears in Alan Sinfield, "Hamlet's Special Providence," *Shakespeare Survey*, vol. 33 (New York: Cambridge University Press, 1980), 89–97.

7. I have chosen Althusser's term because his account of "hailing" stresses the crucial element of recognition in the process of subjection. The paradigmatic example that he uses for this process is the policeman who yells, "Hey you there!" to an individual who recognizes himself in the call and turns around in response. See Louis Althusser, *Lenin and Philosophy and Other Essays*, trans. Ben Brewster (New York: Monthly Review Press, 1971), 127–86, esp. 174. Althusser's technical term for this process is "interpellation," a term whose root in the Latin verb *interpellare* means "to interrupt." By adapting Althusser's term, I want to subsume Althusser's theory of interpellation into an account of subjection that pivots on turns of attention rather than bodies or vision.

8. The difference in responding to the two different calls might be that with the ghost Hamlet is hailed by a feudal ideology of private revenge, whereas with accidents, Hamlet is hailed by a Tudor ideology that is structured around a belief in providence and, as a corollary, obedience to a temporal monarch who is the providential representative. These two ideologies are contrasted in Janis Lull, "Forgetting *Hamlet*: The First Quarto and the Folio," in *The Hamlet First Published (Q1, 1603)*, ed. Thomas Clayton (Newark, N.J.: University of Delaware Press, 1992), 138–39.

9. Because the call is not literal, the turn appears to take place without external prompting—to be willful and self-initiated. This representation of the turn is itself an idealization of the process I am trying to describe, since it circumvents the difficult question of why an individual would feel compelled to respond to an anonymous call. Two essays that foreground this difficulty in Althusser's theory are Judith Butler's, "'Conscience Doth Make Subjects of Us All,'" *Yale French Studies* 88 (1995): 6–26; and Mladen Dolar's, "Beyond Interpellation," *Qui Parle* 6, no. 2 (1993): 75–96. I am interested in this difficulty as well, and want to meet it with an account of inner life that is adapted to the spiritual terms in which that life was understood during this period.

10. In the *Institutes* (Book I, ch. 16, art. 3), Calvin complains that many invoke providence in a sterile or unthinking way, differentiating this reflex from a more sincere recognition of its guiding presence: "For it would be quite insipid to expound the words of the Prophet in the philosophical manner, that God is the prime agent, because he is the principle and cause of all motion; whereas the faithful should rather encourage themselves in the adversity with this consolation, that they suffer no affliction, but by the ordination and command of God" (John Calvin, *Institutes of the Christian Religion*, trans. John Allen, vol. 1 [Philadelphia: Presbyterian Board of Christian Education, 1936], 220–21). The entire chapter revolves around a differentiation between a sleepy form of belief in

God's power and a more impassioned, self-aware form of faith in God's active governance of mundane affairs. On the importance of this theme in Calvin's theology, see William Bouwsma, *John Calvin: A Sixteenth Century Portrait* (Oxford: Oxford University Press, 1988), 174–75.

11. An analysis of these examples and their historical development in Scholastic theology and Calvinism can be found in Chapters 1 and 2.

12. *Institutes,* Book I, ch. 17. art. 1. Allen, trans., 232.

13. Ibid., ch. 16, art. 3. Allen, trans., 220.

14. Ibid., ch. 16, art. 6. Allen, trans., 225.

15. Margo Todd, "Providence, Chance and the New Science in Early Stuart Cambridge," *Historical Journal* 29, no. 3 (1986): 700.

16. "Extra-biblical revelation" is Ronald VanderMolen's phrase. See his "Providence as Mystery, Providence as Revelation: Puritan and Anglican Modifications of John Calvin's Doctrine of Providence," *Church History* 47, no. 1 (1978): 27–47.

17. Thomas Cooper, *Certaine sermons wherin is contained the defense of the gospell nowe preached...* (Londo[n]: Ralphe Newbery, 1580), 164.

18. One theological force behind this burgeoning interest in accidents may have been that, as belief in miracles waned, God's intervention in the world had to become more subtle. Instead of suspending the usual causes in nature for a specific purpose, stopping the sun, for example, or dividing the sea, God could use the "play" or "blind spots" within the world governed by those causes for his own purposes. There is no cause in nature that forbids pirates to meet a ship on its way to England, for example, but there is also no cause that ensures they will not. In the absence of such determining causes, God—not chance or fortune—becomes the final arbiter of what will happen.

19. Keith Thomas, *Religion and the Decline of Magic* (New York: Charles Scribner's Sons, 1971), 93.

20. While Bolton's book is published several decades after *Hamlet* was written, I cite it because he gives an accurate catalogue of the kinds of accidents that would have been considered "judgements" in the sixteenth century as well. (Most critics believe *Hamlet* was written in 1600.) See Robert Bolton, *Some generall directions for a comfortable walking with god: delivered in the lecture at Kettering in Northhamptonshire, with enlargement* (London: Felix Kyngston, 1626), 45. Thomas quotes a later edition. Bolton quotes Romans 13:5 to argue that conformity prompted by conscience is superior to this kind of fearful compliance: "[We] ought to be subject, not onely for wrath, but also for conscience sake" (46).

21. Jean de Chassanion, *The theatre of Gods judgements: or, a collection of histories out of sacred, ecclesiasticall, and prophane authours...* (London: Adam Islip, 1597). VanderMolen contrasts Beard's more aggressive providentialism to that of the Anglican churchman George Hakewill, who criticized those who "are ready to turn every accident to an argument for their own purposes." See VanderMolen, 37.

22. Chassanion, A3r.

23. See Phillip Stubbes, *Two wunderfull and rare examples, of undeferred and present approaching judgement of the Lord our God the one upon a wicked and pernicious blasphemer of the name of God...* (London, 1581), A2v. Blood flowing from the nose would still incite thoughts of guilt later in the seventeenth century. In Webster's *Duchess of Malfi*, for instance, Antonio tries to convince himself that the nosebleed he has while trying to deceive Bosola is a mere accident. "My nose bleeds," he says, adding, "One that were superstitious would count / This ominous, when it merely comes by chance ... Mere accident" (2.3.41–47). See John Webster, *The Duchess of Malfi* in A. K. McIlwraith, ed., *Five Stuart Tragedies* (Oxford: Oxford University Press, 1961), 238.

24. In the 1595 edition of Stubbes *Anatomie of abuses*, he makes this ironic connection between swearing God's blood and bleeding more explicit. See Phil[l]ip Stubbes, *The anatomie of abuses. Containing a description of such notable vices and enormities, as raigne in many countries of the world, but especiallie in this realme of England: together with most fearefull examples of Gods heavie judgements inflicted upon the wicked for the same as well in England of late, as in other places else where...* (London: Richard Johnes, 1595), 97.

25. In the introduction to *Two wunderfull and rare examples*, Stubbes makes reference to the widespread lack of "regard" for God's prescriptions and judgments: "Are not the hearts of men so fast lulled, in the cradle of Securitie, that Pittie is forgotten, Charitie fledde, Mercie exiled, Avarice exalted, good Conscience banished.... Nay, rather the more is the pittie, Exhortations, Examples, Earthquakes, Comettes, fierie Skies, Inundations, Shipwrackes, unnatural birthes, as well in men as beastes, nothing regarded" (A2r–A2v); and in the postscript: "We may beholde (Christian Reader) with no little griefe of minde, the great love of our God, and the lyttle regarde of our selves, his fatherlie motions, and in us no signe of amendment. Referring the innumerable examples, happening not onely to our Fathers, but in our-tyme also."

26. See Samuel Saxey, *A straunge and wonderfull example of the judgement of almighty God, shewed upon two adulterous persons in London, in the parish of S. Brydes, in Fleetestreete, this thurde of Februarie. 1583* (London: [H. Bynneman], 1583), B2r–B3v; and Phillip Stubbes, *The anatomie of abuses: containing, a discoverie, or briefe summarie of such notable vices and imperfections, as now raigne in many countreyes of the world: but (especiallye) in a famous ilande called Ailgna: together, with most fearefull examples of Gods judgements, executed uppon the wicked for the same* ... (Printed at London: By [John Kingston for] Richard Jones, 1583), 109.

27. John Fielde, *A godly exhortation, by occasion of the late judgement of God, shewed at Parris-garden.... Given to all estates for their instruction, concerning the keeping of the Sabboth day* (London, 1583), 2v.

28. Stubbes reports the same incident in the 1595 edition of his *Anatomie of abuses*. He also reports an earlier accident in which theatergoers were thrown out of their seats and injured by an earthquake. See 134–35.

29. *OED*, 8:364–65.

30. Matteo Gribaldi, Edward Aglionby, and Jean Calvin, *A notable and marveilous epistle of the famous doctour, Matthewe Gribalde, Professor of the lawe, in*

the Universitie of Padua: co[n]cernyng the terrible judgemente of God, upon hym that for feare of men, denieth Christ and the knowne veritie: with a preface of Doctor Calvine (London: Henry Denham [and J. Kingston?], 1570).

31. Henry Holland, *The Christian exercise of fasting, private and publike ... Hereunto also are added some meditations on the 1. and 2. chapters of Job, to comfort and instruct all such as be afflicted with any crosse, either inwardly in minde, or outwardly in bodie. By H. Holland, minister and preacher of Gods word* (London: [Orwin], 1596), 159.

32. William Perkins, *A golden chaine: or, The description of theologie, containing the order of the causes of salvation and damnation, according to Gods word. A view whereof is to be seene in the table annexted. Hereunto is adjoyned the order which M. Theodore Beza sed in comforting afflicted consciences* ([Cambridge]: John Legat, 1600), 247.

33. The panoptic ambitions of this scheme should be obvious. See Foucalt's chapter on panopticism in *Discipline and Punish*, trans. Alan Sheridan (New York: Vintage, 1979). In the same chapter, Perkins uses the existence of conscience to prove that providence exists, suggesting that the ability of the individual to bridle sinful action stems from an active awareness of punishments to come. How, he argues, could one fear what is to come if there were no underlying plan that governed future events? See Perkins, 242. The circularity of his argument here is chilling.

34. There are also "deliverances" or "mercies" in which providence accommodates a virtuous activity, but such events are not as popular in the late sixteenth century. This literature really starts to develop in the first decades of the seventeenth century.

35. Enthusiasm for this kind of analysis may have reached its height during the Civil War, but clearly by the end of the sixteenth century accidental events were being recorded and recognized as judgments from God. For an analysis of Interregnum attempts to interpret accidents or "casualties" as signs of God's will, see Barbara Donagan, "Understanding Providence: The Difficulties of Sir William and Lady Waller," *Journal of Ecclesiastical History* 39, no. 3 (1988): 433–44.

36. Terence Cave has studied the use of accidental recognition in *Twelfth Night*, arguing persuasively that the accidental event can both defer and then restore a figurative meaning around which the recognition plot is structured. See Terence Cave, *Recognitions* (Oxford: Clarendon Press, 1988), 276–82.

37. Shakespeare is poking fun at one of the things he must often do as a playwright: relate important information to characters and the audience by means of an artificial device like the set-narration (for example, Egeon at the opening of *The Comedy of Errors*), the dream, the prophecy, or the letter. The most notorious device of the theater, of course, is the deus ex machina: given that the pirate rescue is a *providential* accident, Shakespeare may be nodding at this outdated device as well.

38. Jacques Lezra writes: "By the time of *Hamlet* and *Pericles* pirates are established agents of unexpected intrusion in the plays, figures drawn as it were

proleptically from the Romances to explain discontinuities in the earlier plays." (See Jacques Lezra, *Unspeakable Subjects: The Genealogy of the Event in Early Modern Europe* [Stanford: Stanford University Press, 1997], 270.) Lezra links contemporary commercial and political anxieties about pirates to their function as a figure of "interruption" in Shakespeare's *Measure for Measure*. Both his reading and my own owe something to the work of Richard S. Ide, who argues that "[t]he Shakespearean pirate ... should be understood finally as a metaphor for the intrusion of a just Providence in the affairs of men, indeed as a symbol of God's active government of the world stage." See Richard S. Ide, "Shakespeare and the Pirates," *Iowa State Journal of Research* 58, no. 3 (1984): 317. On Elizabethan and Jacobean policies toward "profiteering"—which ranged from de facto encouragement during the war with Spain to James's proclamation of 1603 revoking any legal protections enjoyed by privateers—see Lezra, 271–73.

39. Perkins, *A golden chaine*, 248. The image runs oddly parallel to the one Claudius uses in his first speech in *Hamlet*, when he is describing his "one dropping eye" (1.2.11).

40. Perkins, 832.

41. Debate about whether or not Hamlet already knows that the two men are watching has turned, in part, on the question of when he makes his entry. Q2, for example, has Hamlet entering just as Polonius is recommending that the two men hide, which would allow Hamlet to see the plot right away. I have chosen the reading in F, and generally agree with Hibbard that Hamlet does not need to know about his audience in advance of this scene. The spontaneous nature of his suspicion seems more in keeping with his character, and certainly makes the scene more dramatic.

42. *OED*, 2:1253–54.

43. If we think of likeness as itself an event, we can find numerous ways in which the more physical model of an accident—an embodied encounter between two agents or objects—can be mapped onto semantic overlappings (this word sounds like that one) or the intersection of memory and theatrical experience (this incident looks like that one). The philosophical analytic of the accident is well suited to these cognitive convergences as well, which are really best described as psychic events.

44. Obviously theatrical consciousness may be distracted by events going on in the audience as well, an important factor in the early modern theater. My theory of distraction could be merged with an analysis of this vector of distraction in the context of performance. The kind of distraction I find modeled in the play and the surrounding literature, however, is of a less literal sort.

45. Stephen Greenblatt articulates the breadth and consequences of this mobility in "The Circulation of Social Energy," in *Shakespearean Negotiations* (Berkeley: University of California Press, 1988), 1–20.

46. Claudius uses this term—providence—to describe his own power as king earlier on (4.1.16–19). On the older, prudential meaning of providence, see Peggy Knapp, *Time Bound Words: Semantic and Social Economies from Chaucer's England to Shakespeare's* (New York: St. Martin's Press, 2000), 114–17.

47. The early modern definition of "device" is as rich and suggestive as that of "conscience," suggesting that it is a faculty of "invention" as well as a plan or stratagem (OED, 3:282–83).

48. The significance of "blasting" and the instability of gunpowder—proverbial in accounts of siege warfare during the period—align this metaphor with the forces of chance.

49. Hibbard makes this point in his introduction to the Oxford edition.

50. Stage directions in F and Q2 are quite different on the exchange. See James L. Jackson, "'They Catch One Another's Rapiers': The Exchange of Weapons in *Hamlet*," *Shakespeare Quarterly* 41, no. 3 (1990): 281–98. If the exchange occurs deliberately (as in a grapple), then Hamlet gains more agency in the providential "accident" than if Laertes simply loses his grip on his weapon.

51. The dormancy of conscience may be an effect of Claudius's failure to give up the benefits of kingship and so obtain some kind of absolution.

52. The process is initiated as soon as Gertrude unexpectedly consumes the poison that was meant for her son. At this point Laertes mentions that it is "almost against my conscience" to follow through with the plan and stab Hamlet with the poison.

53. The importance of occasion and Hamlet's willingness to improvise alongside of chance in this scene allies him with other Renaissance figures who are able to seize "chance" and occasion by the forelock. Like Calvin's providential God or Machiavelli's prince, Hamlet recognizes the optimal occasion for action. On Calvin's proximity to Machiavelli on this point, see William Bouwsma, *John Calvin: A Sixteenth-Century Portrait* (New York: Oxford University Press, 1989), 172.

54. I agree with Greenblatt that the "provisionality" of theatrical performance would not necessarily have been subversive, and conversely, that the hidden order manifest in scripted performance was not necessarily orthodox (*Shakespearean Negotiations*, 18). See also his discussion of the status of theatrical fiction in "Shakespeare and the Exorcists," where he suggests that the illusion on stage never achieves full autonomy in the imagination: "But the audience at a play never absolutely accepts such fictions [as the presence of the Dover cliff in *King Lear*]: we enjoy being brazenly lied to, we welcome for the sake of pleasure what we know to be untrue, but we withhold from the theater the simple assent we grant to everyday reality" (ibid., 119). This distinction between theater and reality is not entirely stable in the early modern context, since a providential "reality" possesses precisely that quality of provisionality associated with the theater.

55. The key word here is temporarily, since as long as providentialists were insisting that the world itself was a theater, the theatrical "illusion" could not entirely empty the ideological scheme of world-as-theater of its power. Recognizing the sheer interpretive power of the providential analogy, I would say that ideology here does not mean simply a structure of domination that depends on a psychic agency for its effects (conscience, regard, the imagination), but also a system that makes the world intelligible. (Debora Shuger offers this

broader definition of ideology in her *Habits of Thought in the English Renaissance* [Berkeley: University of California Press, 1990], 8–9.) Part of the ineluctability of providential interpretation in early modern consciousness stems from the fact that providence as structure-of-intelligibility is itself, also, a form of organized subjection. This kind of overlap does not simply happen, but requires an interested set of writers (like Calvin's English interpreters) to make the theatrical analogy and provide a rationale for its consistent application.

56. The linkage of this kind of experimentation with accident is the subject of the next chapter. From an entirely different perspective, the theater also has a clarifying power in Althusser's essay, in which he points out that his own theory of interpellation is presented in a "little theoretical theater." See Althusser, 174.

57. I find the Derridian vocabulary of deferral and presence, as opposed to the psychoanalytic categories of avowal and disavowal (or remembering and forgetting), quite suggestive for thinking about the status of knowledge in the theater. This kind of deferred knowledge preserves the spectator's state of distraction rather than unifying it in a state of complete absorption (where knowledge of the theater as a performance based on other performances is definitively absent) or total consciousness of artifice (where knowledge of the play's status as an artifact is overwhelmingly present). For an introduction to these terms, see Jacques Derrida, "Différance," in *Margins of Philosophy* (Chicago: University of Chicago Press, 1982), 1–28. I have advocated the provisional or ontologically incomplete nature of all semiotic phenomena in my "Guarantees of the Remarkable," *Qui Parle* 6, no. 2 (1993): 1–40.

58. Hamlet's exclamation when he stabs at the arras, "dead for a ducat," shows that he is aware of the fact that the outcome—like all gambles—is subject to chance. His subsequent remarks confirm that he had hoped to kill Claudius ("I took thee for thy better" [3.4.33]).

59. The accident is coded as artificial when it is delivered in an elegy, a formal piece of verse that stands out from the rest of the play as a kind of miniature of craft. Here perhaps as nowhere else, the lyrical sweep of language makes the accident seem almost inevitable—like a rhyme. This is not the first time Gertrude will disguise a deliberate killing: her description of Hamlet's "mad" lunge at the arras helps to acquit her son of deliberately trying to kill Polonius.

60. In Hamlet's case, the accident that prompts such a withdrawal is the pirate rescue; for Ophelia, it is the death of her father.

61. This form of agency is akin to the reassertion of masculine control of Fortune in Renaissance thought, albeit with a crucial modification: God is the paternal partner in the game rather than the wily female opponent.

Chapter 5: Accident and the Invention of Knowledge

1. The heroic reading of Bacon's modernity is perhaps most powerful in the nineteenth century, but is replaced in the twentieth by the critique of instrumental reason (Horkheimer and Adorno) and feminist analyses of his gendered rhetorics of domination. See for example Max Horkheimer and Theodor W.

Adorno, *Dialectic of Enlightenment,* trans. John Cumming (New York: Continuum, 1995), ch. 1; and Carolyn Merchant, *The Death of Nature: Women, Ecology and the Scientific Revolution* (San Francisco: Harper Collins, 1980), ch. 7.

2. See Niccolo Machiavelli, *The Prince,* ed. Quentin Skinner and Russell Price (Cambridge: Cambridge University Press, 1995), 87. Bacon's will to mastery over nature is apparent in the following passage, taken from his unfinished *Temporis partus masculus,* or *The Masculine Birth of Time*: "I am come in very truth leading to you Nature with all her children to bind her to your service and make her your slave." See Benjamin Farrington's translation in *The Philosophy of Francis Bacon* (Chicago: University of Chicago Press, 1964), 62. Bacon's Latin reads: [S]ed revera naturam cum fetibus suis tibi addicturus et mancipaturus. See Francis Bacon, *The Works of Francis Bacon,* ed. James Spedding, Robert Leslie Ellis, Douglas Denon Heath (New York: Garret Press, 1968), III:528. Bacon's tendency to assimilate the traditional iconography of chance or "occasion" with that of nature is quite striking in the following passage from the *Redargutio philosophiarum*: "[B]elieve that what is said of Time is true of nature. Nature must be taken by the forelock, being bald behind" (Farrington, trans., 130). Spedding et al., eds.: [Q]uin credite mihi, quod de fortuna dici solet id de natura verissimum est, eam a fronte capillatam, ab occipitio calvam esse (583).

3. The translation is that of Peter Urbach and John Gibson, *Novum Organum with Other Parts of the Great Instauration* (Chicago: Open Court, 1994), 45. The Latin text of Fowler's edition reads: Etiam opera, quae jam inventa sunt, casui debentur et experientiae, magis quam scientiis: scientiae enim, quas nunc habemus, nihil aliud sunt quam quaedam concinnationes rerum antea inventarum; non modi inveniendi, aut designationes novorum operum. See *Bacon's Novum Organum,* ed. Thomas Fowler, 2d ed. (Oxford: Clarendon Press, 1889), 195.

4. Urbach et al., trans., 90–91; Fowler, ed., 279: [O]mnia vel traditionum caligini, vel argumentorum vertigini et turbini, vel casus et experientiae vagae et inconditae undis et ambagibus permissa esse.

5. The theme is quite common in the *Novum organum,* although I will cite only a few examples. See his critique of the alchemists as making their discoveries through "chance, incidentally, or by some variation of experiments" [*tanquam fortuito et obiter, aut per experimentorum quandam variationem*] (Urbach et al., trans., 83; Fowler, ed., 266); a description of how the mechanical arts have made their discoveries *per occasiones obvias et contemplationes incurrentes* (Fowler, ed., 285; Urbach et al. translate as "chance ideas," 94); his complaint that the arts of discovery now in use discourage industry in the sciences, which in turn "throws away the chances that experience itself might yield" [*ipsius experientiae aleas abjiciat*] (Urbach et al., trans., 98; Fowler, ed., 289); his comment that the previously unthinkable correspondence between the navigational compass and the stars was not discovered by philosophy or arts of reasoning, "but by chance and favorable circumstances" [*sed casu et per occasionem*] (Urbach et al., trans., 114; Fowler, ed., 314).

6. See *Francis Bacon: A Critical Edition of the Major Works,* ed. Brian Vickers

(New York: Oxford University Press, 1996), 198. Subsequent references to this work appear parenthetically in the text.

7. Bacon's interest in discovering "rules" for deliberate action is described in Antonio Pérez-Ramos, *Francis Bacon's Idea of Science and the Maker's Knowledge Tradition* (Oxford: Clarendon Press, 1988), ch. 10.

8. Studies of Bacon's *ars inveniendi* tend to relate it, with good reason, to the late Renaissance arts of dialectical and rhetorical invention. Lisa Jardine, for example, argues that Bacon's theory of invention is best understood in relation to dialectical methods popular in humanist reforms of the late sixteenth century. See her *Francis Bacon: Discovery and the Art of Discourse* (Cambridge: Cambridge University Press, 1974). My own discussion of the invention of knowledge will focus not on the schemes used for such invention but the epistemological conditions that those schemes satisfy.

9. Urbach et al., trans., 112–13; Fowler, ed., 312: Atque de desperatione tollenda et spe facienda, ex praeteriti temporis erroribus valere jussis aut rectificatis, jam dictum est. Videndum autem et si quae alia sint quae spem faciant. Illud vero occurrit; si hominibus non quaerentibus, et aliud agentibus, multa utilia, tanquam casu quodam aut per occasionem, inventa sint; nemini dubium esse posse, quin iisdem quaerentibus et hoc agentibus, idque via et ordine, non impetu et desultorie, longe plura detegi necesse sit.

10. Urbach et al., trans., 91; Fowler, ed., 280: Restat experientia mera: quae, si occurrat, casus; s[i] quaesita sit, experimentum nominatur.

11. In the last two decades, intellectual historians have begun to emphasize Bacon's preference for knowledge gained in unusual circumstances. See, for example, Katharine Park and Lorraine Daston, "Unnatural Conceptions: The Study of Monsters in Sixteenth- and Seventeenth-Century France and England," *Past and Present* 92 (1981): 20–54; and William Eamon, *Science and the Secrets of Nature* (Princeton: Princeton University Press, 1994), ch. 8.

12. See Farrington, 67. Bacon's Latin reads: [U]bi sane magna mentiendi reciprocatione inter se conciliati largas ubique spes ostentant, et per experientiae quidem devia vagi, in quaedam utilia, casu non ductu, quandoque impinguntur. See Spedding et al., eds., III:533–34.

13. I have modified Farrington's translation (71) to highlight Bacon's qualification of chance and Spedding's comments on this passage. Spedding et al., eds., III:538: Sus rostro si forte humi A literam impresserit, num propterea suspicabere integram tragoediam, veluti literam unam, ab ea posse describi? Longe alia est ratio (fili) veritatis quae est ex scientiae analogia, alia quae ex idoli sectione enuntiatur. Illa constans et quota gemina, haec discors et solitaria. Quod etiam in operibus fit. Pulvis tormentorum si ductu, non casu (ut loquuntur) et impactu inventum fuisset, non solitarium, sed cum multa inventorum nobilium (quae sub eundem meridianum cadunt) frequentia prodiisset. (As Spedding notes, the phrase "ex idoli sectione enuntiatur" suggests something discovered by the cutting or intersection of a baseless hypothesis with the truth. There may be some overlap here between the notion of intersection and the Scholastic notion of accident as the crossing of causal lines.)

14. The image is taken directly from Cicero's *De divinatione* 1.13, a passage in which Quintus condemns the view that artistic images (sculptures and painting) could be perfected by *casus*. At the end of the passage, Quintus argues that "it is undeniably true that no perfect imitation of a thing was ever made by chance." See Cicero, *De divinatione*, trans. William Falconer (Cambridge, Mass.: Harvard University Press, 1974), 250–51: Sus rostro si humi A litteram impresserit, num propterea suspicari poteris Andromacham Ennii ab ea posse describi ... Sic enim se profecto res habet, ut numquam perfecte veritatem casus imitetur. (I will comment on this connection between chance and artistry below.)

15. Farrington, 73. Spedding et al., eds., III:591: [E]aque ipsa [inventa hominum] quae hactenus humana exhibuit industria, Philosophiae haud attribui.

16. Farrington, 73. Spedding et al., eds., III:591: Casum, authorem rerum proculdubio utilem; sed qui per longas ambages et circuitus donaria sua in homines spargat.

17. Farrington, 91. Spedding et al., eds., III:609: Restare experientiam meram; quae, si occurrit, casus, si quaesita sit, Experimentum nominatur ... Quin et eos qui in aliqua natura vel operatione per multam et erraticam quandam experimentorum variationem revelanda et in lucem educenda sedulo occupati sunt, aut attonitos stare, aut vertiginosos circumire, aliquando gestientes, aliquando confusos, atque semper invenire quod ulterius quaerant.

18. The alchemists were particularly good at producing these unusual situations, but did so blindly. Bacon writes in *NO*, Book I, Aphorism 73: "It is true that alchemists have some achievements from their labours, but these came by chance, incidentally, or by some variation of experiments, such as mechanics are accustomed to make, and not from any art or theory" (Urbach et al., trans., 83). The Latin: At Chymicorum industria nonnulla peperit; sed tanquam fortuito et obiter, aut per experimentorum quandam variationem (ut mechanici solent), non ex arte aut theoria aliqua (Fowler, ed., 266).

19. See Pérez-Ramos, 68–96, esp. 91.

20. Rossi surveys the alchemical and hermetic traditions engaged by the Baconian program. See Paolo Rossi, *Francis Bacon: From Magic to Science*, trans. Sacha Rabinovitch (London: Routledge & Kegan Paul, 1968), chs. 2–3.

21. Graham Rees has extended the range of Bacon's intellectual resources even further by pointing out the remarkably eclectic nature of Bacon's works on specific natural phenomena (for example, on the heavens, on density and rarity, and on animal spirit). See *The Oxford Francis Bacon*, ed. Graham Rees (Oxford: Clarendon Press, 1996), VI:xxxvi–lxix.

22. See Julian Martin, *Francis Bacon, the State, and the Reform of Natural Philosophy* (Cambridge: Cambridge University Press, 1992), 167. Martin's work is building upon that of a number of previous scholars. See, for example, Paul Kocher, "Francis Bacon on the Science of Jurisprudence," *Journal of the History of Ideas* 18 (1957): 3–26; and Kenneth William Cardwell, "Francis Bacon, Inquisitor," in *Francis Bacon's Legacy of Texts*, ed. William A. Sessions (New York: AMS Press, 1990), 269–89.

23. See Lisa Jardine, "*Experientia Literata* or *Novum Organum*," in Sessions, ed., 47–67.

24. On the epistemological modesty of probabilist epistemologies in seventeenth-century England, see Barbara Shapiro, *Probability and Certainty in Seventeenth-Century England* (Princeton: Princeton University Press, 1983).

25. Urbach et al., trans., 138; Fowler, ed., 351–52. Elsewhere in this aphorism, Bacon refers to the simple natures in bodies as being conjoined in a structure [*collegiatas et in fabrica*], so that the body itself is a troop or collection of simple natures [*turmam sive conjugationem naturarum simplicium*].

26. Presumably, the definitions of the simple natures may also be refined in this process, but Bacon does not give detailed instructions on how to do this.

27. Book II, Aphorisms 11–13. See Urbach et al., trans., 144–68; and Fowler, ed., 360–95.

28. Book II, Aphorisms 15 and 18. See Urbach et al., trans., 168, 171; and Fowler ed., 395–96, 400–402, respectively.

29. Bacon proposes a total of nine further helps for induction in Book II, Aphorism 21, but covers only the first in the remaining aphorisms. These are the twenty-seven classes of "Prerogative Instances," or *Praerogativas Instantiarum,* that allow the simple natures to appear more readily. The Prerogative Instances appear to be a series of *topoi* that allow for the invention (in the sense of discovery) of alternative instances which might serve as the basis for further refinement and exclusions.

30. Urbach et al., trans., 173; Fowler, ed., 403.

31. Maxwell Primack, "Outline of a Reinterpretation of Francis Bacon's Philosophy," *Journal of the History of Philosophy* 5, no. 2 (1967): 132.

32. Urbach et al., trans., 138; Fowler, ed., 351: Eadem enim est ratio generandi naturam unam aliquam simplicem, et plures; nisi quod arctetur magis et restringatur homo in operando, si plures requirantur, propter difficultatem tot naturas coadunandi; quae non facile conveniunt, nisi per vias naturae tritas et ordinarias. Utcunque tamen dicendum est, quod iste modus operandi (qui naturas intuetur simplices, licet in corpore concreto) procedat ex iis, quae in natura sunt constantia et aeterna et catholica, et latas praebeat potentiae humanae vias, quales (ut nunc sunt res) cogitatio humana vix capere aut repraesentare possit.

33. See for example Horst Brederkamp, *The Lure of Antiquity and the Cult of the Machine*, trans. Allison Brown (Princeton: Markus Wiener Publishers, 1995), 66–67; Lorraine Daston, "Baconian Facts, Academic Civility, and the Prehistory of Objectivity," *Annals of Scholarship* 8, no. 3–4 (1991): 337–63, esp. 344; and Park and Daston, 43–51.

34. See Paula Findlen, "Jokes of Nature and Jokes of Knowledge: The Playfulness of Scientific Discourse in Early Modern Europe," *Renaissance Quarterly* 43 (1990): 292–331, esp. 318. Findlen argues that Continental naturalists in the sixteenth and seventeenth centuries were quite self-conscious about the way in which "jokes of nature" oscillated between the categories of the natural and the made.

35. See H. W. Janson, "The 'Image Made by Chance' in Renaissance Thought," in *De Artibus Opuscula XL: Essays in Honor of Erwin Panofsky*, ed. Millard Meiss (New York: New York University Press, 1961), 254–66; and Findlen, 297: "[T]he post-classical conception of lusus . . . described images made by chance." A summary of Greek views on nature as artist or craftsman appears in Friedrich Solmsen, "Nature as Craftsman in Greek Thought," *Journal of the History of Ideas* 24, no. 4 (1963): 473–96.

36. The word "deflexion" here resonates with a similar use of the word in *Valerius Terminus of the Interpretation of Nature*, in which Bacon describes "Anticipation" as "a deflexion or declination by accident." See Spedding et al., eds., III:251.

37. Janson, 260–61.

38. See footnotes 13 and 14 above for a comparison of the two texts.

39. The Singular Instances, by contrast (elephants among quadrupeds, or the letter S, which is unusually able to combine with consonants), are examples of unusual combinations or degrees that do not result from a chance deviation.

40. Urbach et al., trans., 197; Fowler, ed., 444: Si enim deprehendatur semel natura in variatione sua . . . expeditum erit eo deducere naturam per artem quo per casum aberraverit . . . cum errores ex una parte monstrent et aperiant viam ad errores et deflexiones undequaque.

41. Urbach et al., trans., 199–200; Fowler, ed., 447: Quocirca omnia inventa, quae censeri possunt magis nobilia (si animum advertas), in lucem prodiere, nullo modo per pusillas enucleationes et extensiones artium, sed omnino per casum. Nihil autem repraesentat aut anticipat casum (cujus mos est ut tantum per longa saecula operetur), praeter inventionem formarum.

42. Urbach et al., trans., 114; Fowler, ed., 314: Itaque sperandum omnino est, esse adhuc in naturae sinu multa excellentis usus recondita, quae nummal cum jam inventis cognationem habent aut parellelismum, sed omnino sita sunt extra vias phantasiae; quae tamen adhuc inventa non sunt; quae proculdubio per multos saeculorum circuitus et ambages et ipsa quandoque prodibunt, sicut illa superiora prodierunt; sed per viam, quam nunc tractamus, propere et subito et simul repraesentari et anticipari possunt.

43. Farrington, 48.

44. For a useful summary of Bacon's changing views on the allegorical interpretation of fables, his sources, and the possible philosophical meaning of his writings that treat of ancient myths, see Rossi, ch. 3, esp. 88–101.

45. Spedding et al., eds., VI:708, 636: [C]um Ceres moesta et ob raptam Proserpinam indignata se abscondisset, atque dii omnes ad eam investigandam magnopere incubuissent, et se per varias vias dispertiti essent; Pani solummodo ex felicitate quadam contigisse, ut inter venandum eam inveniret et indicaret.

46. Ibid., 713, 640: [Ne] rerum utilium ad vitam et cultum inventio, qualis fuit segetum, a philosophiis abstractis, tanquam diis majoribus, expectetur, licet totis viribus in illud ipsum incumbant; sed tantummodo a Pane, id est, expe-

rientia sagaci et rerum mundi notitia universali, quae etiam casu quodam ac veluti inter venandum in huiusmodi inventa incidere solet.

47. William Eamon is correct in suggesting that Pan's travels are guided by *mêtis*—a hunter's instincts and cunning (285–91). Bacon still feels compelled, however, to recognize that chance of some kind is involved in *Experientia Literata*. On *mêtis* and the "venatic method," see Carlo Ginzburg's "Clues: Roots of an Evidential Paradigm," in *Clues, Myths and the Historical Method*, trans. John and Anne Tedeschi (Baltimore: Johns Hopkins University Press, 1989), 96–125.

48. *De augmentis scientiarum*, in Spedding et al., eds., I:623, IV:413.

49. Ibid., I:624, IV:413.

50. Ibid., I:627, IV:416.

51. Elsewhere in *De augmentis*, Bacon notes that in the past humans have been beholden to chance for the inventions of medical and military arts (I:618–19, IV:408–9).

52. Ibid., IV:420. The Latin: Hic vero experimentandi modus plane irrationalis est, et quasi furiosus; cum aliquid experiri velle animum subeat, not quia aut ratio aut aliquod aliud experimentum te ad illud deducat, sed prorsus quia similis res adhuc nunquam tentata fuit. Haud tamen scio, an in hac ipsa re (de qua nunc agimus) non aliquid magni lateat; si, inquam, omnem lapidem in natura moveas. Magnalia enim naturae fere extra vias tritas et orbitas notas jacent, ut etiam absurditas rei aliquando juvet. At si ratio simul comitetur; id est, ut et manifestum sit simile experimentum nunquam tentatum fuisse, et tamen causa subsit magna cur tentetur; tum vero haec res ex optimis est, et plane sinus naturae excutit (I:632).

53. For an account of the social and literary conventions that assured this space, in addition to the conditions created by the instrument itself, see Steven Shapin and Simon Shaffer, *Leviathan and the Airpump: Hobbes, Boyle, and the Experimental Life* (Princeton: Princeton University Press, 1985).

54. Robert Boyle, "An Examen of Mr. T. Hobbes his Dialogus Physicus de Natura Aëris," in *The Works of the Honourable Robert Boyle*, 5 vols. (London, 1744), I:123.

55. Blumenberg makes the following observation about the epistemological power of accident in Bacon's method: "So much had remained concealed from the human spirit throughout many centuries and was discovered neither by philosophy nor by the faculty of reason but rather by accident and favorable opportunity, because it was all too different and distant from what was familiar, so that no preconception (*praenotio aliqua*) could lead one to it. Thus one may hope that nature conceals in its womb still more, of greater importance, which lies entirely outside the familiar paths of the power of imagination (*extra vias phantasiae*) and which one can only be sure of finding through the systematization of accident." Hans Blumenberg, *The Legitimacy of the Modern Age*, trans. Robert M. Wallace (Cambridge, Mass.: MIT Press, 1983), 389.

56. See *Discourse on the Method* in *The Philosophical Writings of Descartes*, trans. John Cottingham et al., 2 vols. (Cambridge: Cambridge University Press, 1985), I:120. On the dynamics of intrigue in Tudor England, see Lacey Baldwin

Smith, *Treason in Tudor England: Politics and Paranoia* (Princeton: Princeton University Press, 1986); and Patricia Parker, "*Othello* and *Hamlet*: Dilation, Spying, and the 'Secret Place' of Woman," *Representations* 44 (1993): 60–95.

57. Urbach et al., trans., 108; Fowler, ed., 304: Quemadmodum enim in civilibus ingenium cujusque, et occultus animi affectuumque sensus, melius elicitur, cum quis in perturbatione ponitur, quam alias: simili modo, et occulta naturae magis se produnt per vexationes artium, quam cum cursu suo meant.

58. On the relationship between judicial torture and Bacon's method, see Elizabeth Hansen, "Torture and Truth in Renaissance England," *Representations* 34 (1991): 53–84; and Julian Martin, *Francis Bacon, the State, and the Reform of Natural Philosophy* (Cambridge: Cambridge University Press, 1992), 166. On the theory and practice of judicial torture more generally, see John H. Langbein, *Torture and the Law of Proof: Europe and England in the Ancien Regime* (Chicago: University of Chicago Press, 1977).

59. See Cicero, *De inventione, De optimo genere oratorum, Topica*, trans. H. M. Hubbell (Cambridge, Mass.: Harvard University Press, 1976), 440–41.

60. Examples of accidental discoveries of plots in plays include Shakespeare's *Othello* (which I discussed in Chapter 2) and his *All Is True (Henry VIII)*, in which a plot against Henry is established beyond doubt when letters detailing the plot are accidentally delivered to the king. Another example from Webster's *White Devil*: Brachiano's sudden belief that Vittoria is a whore when he intercepts Francisco's letter. See *Othello*, 3.3.33; and *All Is True* (*Henry VIII*), 3.2.29–36, 3.2.200–228, in William Shakespeare, *The Complete Works*, ed. S. Wells and G. Taylor (Oxford: Clarendon Press, 1988), 834, 1210–12; and *The White Devil* (4.2), in Gamini Salgado, ed., *Three Jacobean Tragedies* (London: Penguin Books, 1979), 203–7. The plans of Dr. William Parry, executed for plotting against the queen in 1585, were said to have been revealed providentially by a "sudden interruption of his endeavor." (The figure of providence may have belied a more immediate reliance on a network of spies for sudden interruptions.) See Lowell Gallagher, *Medusa's Gaze: Casuistry and Conscience in the Renaissance* (Stanford: Stanford University Press, 1991), 96–97.

61. This idea of practiced ease, or *sprezzatura*, appears in Baldesar Castiglione's *The Book of the Courtier* (Garden City, N.Y.: Doubleday, 1959), 43.

62. James Kinneavy suggests that one source of the Renaissance interest in *kairos* or occasion was Cicero's ethics and rhetoric, both of which stressed propriety. See his "*Kairos*: A Neglected Concept in Classical Rhetoric," in *Rhetoric and Praxis: The Contribution of Classical Rhetoric to Practical Reasoning*, ed. Jean Dietz Moss (Washington: Catholic University of America Press, 1986), 82.

63. Machiavelli's variable position on the scope of Fortune's power is related to humanist, medieval and classical views in Pitkin, ch. 6, esp. 143 and 149.

64. An absurdity in one intellectual system—the idea that an accident might reveal something universal, which would have been rejected in Scholastic thought—becomes a starting point for another. Amos Funkenstein saw this kind of reversal as a recurring feature in intellectual history. See his *Theology and the Scientific Imagination* (Princeton: Princeton University Press, 1986), 14.

65. Here I am in fundamental agreement with Evelyn Fox Keller's suggestion that Bacon's model for knowing nature was, metaphorically speaking, hermaphroditic. See her *Reflections on Gender and Science* (New Haven: Yale University Press, 1985), 42. Like his theory of knowing, Bacon's theory of action was similarly divided between apparently contradictory—and historically conventional—postures of masculine deliberation and female variability.

Chapter 6: Wonders Taken for Signs

1. The details of my narration here are taken from contemporary accounts of the event discussed below, many of which are assembled in the bibliographical essay by Arthur Freeman, "*The fatal vesper* and *The doleful evensong:* Claim-Jumping in 1623," *Library* 22, no. 2 (1967): 128–35. Theodorus Harmsen also examines the event in his introduction to John Gee's *Foot out of the Snare* (Theodorus Harmsen, *John Gee's* Foot out of the Snare *[1624]* [Nijmegen: Cicero Press, 1992], 49–59).

2. Sidney writes, for example: "So no doubt the philosopher, with his learned definition, be it of virtue, vices, matters of public policy or private government, replenisheth the memory with many infallible grounds of wisdom, which, notwithstanding, lie dark before the imaginative and judging power if they be not illuminated or figured forth by the speaking picture of poesy." See Philip Sidney, *An Apology for Poetry* (Indianapolis: Bobbs-Merrill, 1970), 28. Sidney assumes that there is a didactic use for poetry, and in doing so echoes a teleological strain in Aristotelian poetics, where plot is assumed to have a purposive unity similar to that of a biological system. On the biological bias in Aristotelian poetics, see Elizabeth Belfiore, *Tragic Pleasures: Aristotle on Plot and Emotion* (Princeton: Princeton University Press, 1992), 113–14.

3. In reflecting on the accident's "aesthetic" value, I am trying to show how different this early modern poetic sensibility was from the one Kant proposed in *The Critique of Judgment* I:5: "Taste is the faculty of judging of an object or a method of representing it by means of delight or aversion apart from any interest" (Immanuel Kant, *The Critique of Judgment*, trans. James Creed Meredith [Oxford: Clarendon Press, 1989], 50). Judgments about the tragic significance of Blackfriars were *both* poetic and interested.

4. The process of the naturalization of marvels is described in Katherine Park and Lorraine Daston, "Unnatural Conceptions: The Study of Monsters in Sixteenth- and Seventeenth-Century France and England," *Past and Present* 92 (1981): 20–54. They have since altered their position, however, arguing that naturalistic modes of interpreting marvels coexisted with portentous ones throughout the sixteenth and seventeenth centuries. See Lorraine Daston and Katharine Park, *Wonders and the Order of Nature: 1150–1750* (New York: Zone Books, 1998), ch. 5, hereafter cited as *WO*. Ottavia Niccoli describes how monstrous births gradually lost their value as prophetic signs in Italy in the mid-sixteenth century in *Prophecy and People in Renaissance Italy*, trans. Lydia G. Cochrane (Princeton: Princeton University Press, 1990), 189–90.

5. *WO*, 189.

6. See *The Advancement of Learning*, Book II, in Brian Vickers, ed., *Francis Bacon: A Critical Edition of the Major Works* (Oxford: Oxford University Press, 1996), 195, 199.

7. Daston and Park point to monsters as a paradigmatic case "for the cooperation of primary and secondary causes" (192). Elsewhere, they suggest that the early modern category of the "preternatural" was at times interchangeable with the "accidental" (121). Similarly, in "Baconian Facts, Academic Civility and the Prehistory of Objectivity," Daston argues that anomalous phenomena were ontologically understood as the "product of coincidences and variability" (346). The assumption in theories of providence that primary and secondary causes could cooperate is noted in Keith Thomas, *Religion and the Decline of Magic* (New York: Charles Scribner's Sons, 1971), 80, 91. Preternatural occurrences could also be naturalized by attributing them to errors of perception—one of Nicole Oresme's strategies.

8. John Calvin, *Institutes of the Christian Religion*, trans. John Allen, vol. 1 (Philadelphia: Presbyterian Board of Christian Education, 1936), 26–28.

9. Vickers, ed., 177. A larger intellectual context for this conflict over miracles can be found in medieval debates between voluntarists like William of Ockham, who argued that every aspect of creation was contingent upon God's will, and rationalists like Thomas Aquinas, who argued for the necessary (and so rule-bound) connection between created substances. The opposition and its development in the mechanical philosophies of René Descartes and Pierre Gassendi are described in Margaret J. Osler, *Divine Will and the Mechanical Philosophy: Gassendi and Descartes on Contingency and Necessity in the Created World* (Cambridge: Cambridge University Press, 1994), ch. 1 et passim.

10. *Metaphysics*, 983a 14–21. See Aristotle, *The Complete Works of Aristotle*, ed. Jonathan Barnes, vol. 2 (Princeton: Princeton University Press, 1984), 1555.

11. Book 21, chs. 4–7. For Augustine, wonder can proceed from both a human ignorance of causes and a specifically miraculous intervention into the mundane world: neither is ruled out. See Augustine, *City of God*, trans. Henry Bettenson, ed. David Knowles (Baltimore: Penguin Classics, 1976), 968–79, esp. 977, on God's power to accomplish the "impossible."

12. Caroline Walker Bynum, "Presidential Address: Wonder," *American Historical Review* 102, no. 1 (1997): 1–26.

13. See Bacon, *Works*, II:102. This development is discussed in Park and Daston, "Unnatural Conceptions," 43–51.

14. See *The Philosophical Writings of Descartes*, trans. John Cottingham et al., vol. 1 (Cambridge: Cambridge University Press, 1985), 53. Bynum points out that the physiological account was implicit in Albert's commentary on Aristotle's *Metaphysics*. Stephen Greenblatt, on the other hand, emphasizes the cognitive rather than physiological nature of Descartes's theory. See Stephen Greenblatt, *Marvelous Possessions* (Chicago: University of Chicago Press, 1991), 19. For Greenblatt, wonder is an exalted form of attention that stands in opposi-

tion to resonance, where the latter is understood as a diffusion of consciousness outside the formal boundaries of a given artifact or context. (See Stephen Greenblatt, *Learning to Curse: Essays in Early Modern Culture* [New York: Routledge, 1990], 170.) On this model, the affective and cognitive experience of resonance is like the dilation of an iris, while wonder is its constriction.

15. This sequence of wondering and then knowing is also implicit in the Cartesian scheme, as Philip Fisher points out. Fisher acknowledges the limits of this scheme: it does not apply to what he calls "demotic" wonder at monsters, prodigies and the like. See Philip Fisher, "The Poetics of Wonder," in *Meaning in the Visual Arts: Views from the Outside*, ed. Irving Lavin (Princeton: Institute for Advanced Study, 1993), 175–93.

16. An exhaustive survey of the four senses of Scripture appears in Henri de Lubac, *Medieval Exegesis*, trans. Mark Sebanc (Grand Rapids, Mich.: W. B. Eerdmans, 1998). A much more focused discussion appears in Georges Didi-Huberman, *Fra Angelico: Dissemblance and Figuration*, trans. Jane Marie Todd (Chicago: University of Chicago Press, 1995), 40–41. Didi-Huberman quotes William of Saint-Thierry to the effect that anagogy aims toward the *osculum aeternitatis*—the kiss of eternity. See also Steven Ozment, *The Age of Reform, 1250–1550: An Intellectual and Religious History of Late Medieval and Reformation Europe* (New Haven: Yale University Press, 1980), 66.

17. Like so many of the critical terms in this book, Frye's use of anagogy is idiosyncratic. See Northrop Frye, *Anatomy of Criticism: Four Essays* (Princeton: Princeton University Press, 1990), 119–28, esp. 124.

18. Harmsen points out that Gee may have been at the gathering as an informer (53). It is also possible that he wanted to waver publicly about his faith to increase the propaganda value of his subsequent reconversion.

19. Richard Hord, *Black-Fryers* (London: J. Marriot and J. Grismand, 1625).

20. [Thomas Goad], *The dolefull even-song, or a true particular and impartiall narration of that fearefull and sudden calamity, which befell the preacher Mr. Drury a Jesuite, and the greater part of his Auditory by the downefall of the floore at an assembly in the Black-Friers on Sunday the 26 of Octob. last, in the after noone* (London: John Haviland, 1623).

21. [Goad], D2v. Although the adjectives he uses to describe the sight stop short of wonder, his repeated references to the "tragicall" nature of the spectacle seem to imply it.

22. [John Wilson], *A song, or story, for the lasting rememberance of divers famous works, which God hath done in our time* (London, 1626), 35.

23. [Goad], E2r. This reference to a ten-year-old girl's reaction also appears in *The fatall vesper*, which I discuss below. The child seems to be a trustworthy reporter and interpreter of the event because her reaction is, presumably, untouched by sectarian zeal.

24. *Something written by occasion of that fatall and memorable accident in the Blacke Friers on Sonday, being the 26. of October 1623. stilo antiquo, and the 5. of November stilo novo, or Romano* ([London]: 1623), 5. Freeman (132–33) points out that Goad may have stalled publication of *Something written*—which he could

do because he was a censor—so that his own report could incorporate some of its details and, more important, so that his pamphlet might appear first.

25. The debate over whether or not the event was a providential accident or "meere accident" appeals to a distinction that Perkins made between "chance" and "meere chance" at the turn of the century in *A golden chaine*. See William Perkins, *A golden chain* (Cambridge: John Legat, 1600), 243. Perkins associates mere chance with a complete absence of cause, whereas chance covers events with hidden causes.

26. W. C., *The fatall vesper, or A true and punctuall relation of that lamentable and fearefull accident, hapning on Sunday in the afternoone being the 26. of October last, by the fall of a roome in the Black-Friers, in which were assembled many people at a sermon, which was to be preached by Father Drurie a Jesuite. Together with the names and number of such persons as therin unhappily perished, or were miraculously preserved* (London: John Haviland, 1623), D3v, F4v.

27. The question of why certain people were killed because of *where* they were standing is particularly troubling to survivors. John Gee, for example, survived the fall when all of those around him died. "Surely," he writes of his experience, "when I record this common down-fall, which wounded others unto death, and mee but unto affright, I cannot but strike my brest, and look up into heaven, or rather with the Publican, down to earth, and say, What was there, or is there in mee, miserable man, that the hand of God should strike so many on my right hand and left, and yet overpasse mee?" See John Gee, *The foot out of the snare with a detection of sundry late practices and impostures of the priests and Jesuits in England. Whereunto is added a catalogue of such books as in this authors knowledge have been vented within two yeres past in London, by the priests and their agents* (London: H. L., 1624), 6.

28. Freeman notes contemporary suspicion that the author was a Catholic sympathizer (129).

29. [John Floyd], *A word of comfort. Or A discourse concerning the late lamentable accident of the fall of a roome, at a Catholike sermon, in the Black-friars at London, wherwith about fourscore persons were oppressed. Written for the comfort of Catholiks, and information of Protestants, by I. R. p.* ([Saint-Omer: English College Press], 1623).

30. Elsewhere Floyd notes that accidents can sometimes be produced by the devil, who is given God's permission to act in this way or that; the result is that accidents are situated in the realm of the mundane. See Floyd, 17.

31. On the growth of a literate reading public in London during the seventeenth century, see Tessa Watt, *Cheap Print and Popular Piety, 1550–1640* (Cambridge: Cambridge University Press, 1991), 7; and Nigel Wheale, *Writing and Society: Literacy, Print and Politics in Britain 1590–1660* (New York: Routledge, 1999), 13–15.

32. As far as the subject is concerned, accounts of the Blackfriars accident have an early analog in John Field's *A godly exhortation* (1583), which describes the fall of a scaffolding on Londoners who were watching a bear-baiting on the Sabbath. I discuss this account in Chapter 4.

33. *Lamentable newes out of Monmouthshire in Wales. Contayning, the wonderfull and most fearefull accidents of the great overflowing of waters in the saide countye, drowning infinite numbers of cattell of all kinds, as sheepe, oxen, kine and horses, with others: together with the losse of many men, women and children, and the subversion of xxvi parishes in January last 1607* (London: [Edward Allde], 1607), B4v.

34. *More strange newes: of wonderfull accidents hapning by the late overflowings of waters, in Summerset-shire, Gloucestershire, Norfolke, and other places of England: with a true relation of the townes names that are lost, and the number of persons drowned, with other reports of accidents that were not before discovered: happening about Bristow and Barstable* (London: W[illiam] J[aggard], 1607), B2v.

35. *Lamentable newes, shewing the wonderfull deliverance of Maister Edmond Pet sayler, and maister of a ship, dwelling in Seething Lane in London, neere Barking Church. With other strange things lately hapned concerning these great windes and tempestuous weather, both at sea and land* (London: T. C., 1613), in Joseph Arnold Foster, ed., *Reprints of English Books, 1475–1700,* vol. 1 (Claremont, Calif.: 1948).

36. *Novum organum,* Book I, Aphorism 46. The passage from *Novum Organum with Other Parts of The Great Instauration,* trans. Peter Urbach and John Gibson (Chicago: Open Court, 1994), 57, reads: So it was a good answer made by that man who, on being shown a picture hanging in a temple of those who, having taken their vows, had escaped shipwreck, was asked whether he did not now recognize the power of the gods. He asked in turn: "But where are the pictures of those who perished after taking their vows?" Urbach et al. note that this example is patterned on another from Cicero.

37. The topic of fire in London history is a massive one; accordingly, my remarks here should not be construed as synoptic.

38. *Newes from France. A true relation of the great losses which happened by the lamentable accident of fire in the citie of Paris, the 24. day of October last past, 1621. which burnt downe the Merchants Bridge, the Changers Bridge, and divers houses neere unto them. Together with the speedy diligence used by the Duke De Monbason, governour of the said towne, for the quenching thereof. Also a decree made in the Court of Parliament in Paris, whereby an order is taken for providing for the merchants that have lost their goods by the sayd fire, and to prevent the like mischance in time to come. Translated according to the French copie, printed at Paris* (London: [G. Purslowe], 1621), Bv.

39. *A relation of the most lamentable burning of the cittie of Corke, in the west of Ireland, in the province of Monster, by thunder and lightning. With other most dolefull and miserable accidents, which fell out the last of May 1622 after the prodigious battell of the birds called stares, which fought strangely over and near that citie the 12. and 14. of May 1621* (London: I. D., 1622).

40. Ibid., "To the courteous reader," A3r. For the full account, see *The wonderfull battell of starelings: fought at the citie of Corke in Ireland, the 12. and 14. of October last past. 1621. As it hath been credibly enformed by diverse noblemen and others of the said kingdome...* (London: 1622) in Foster, ed. Such a marvel had been described before in volume six of the *Histoires prodigiueses,* cited in Jean Céard, *La*

Nature et les prodiges: L'Insolité au XVI siècle, en France (Genève: Librarie Droz, 1977), 334.

41. William Gouge, *Gods three arrowes, plague, famine, sword, in three treatises* (London: George Miller, 1631). Gouge was a Puritan minister at St. Anne's, Blackfriars, whose sermon was interrupted by the downfall. It was Gouge who had the timber under the flooring investigated, having heard Catholic rumors that it had been tampered with. See Harmsen, 54.

42. The growth of cheap religious print literature in the early seventeenth century would have included accident literature as well. Watt describes the expansion of this inexpensive form of religious literature and a corresponding "marketplace theology" in *Cheap Print and Popular Piety*, 303–20.

43. See Daniel Defoe, *Robinson Crusoe*, ed. Michael Shinagel (New York: W. W. Norton, 1994), 58–60, 64–67. On Defoe's use of retrospective, postconversion narration, see Michael McKeon, *The Origins of the English Novel, 1600–1740* (Baltimore: Johns Hopkins University Press, 1987), 317.

44. The prohibition against speculating on final causes in natural philosophy appears in the *Novum organum*, Book II, Aphorism 2. See Urbach et al., trans., 134–35; and *Bacon's Novum Organum*, trans. Thomas Fowler, 2d ed. (Oxford: Clarendon Press, 1889), 345–47. Bacon's remark about God's "politique" providence appears in Book II of *The Advancement of Learning*. See *Francis Bacon: A Critical Edition of the Major Works*, ed. Brian Vickers (New York: Oxford University Press, 1996), 199.

45. Ibid., 186.

46. Bacon is noticeably less restrictive in his treatment of accidental occurrences in civil history. See John Tinkler, "Bacon and History," in *The Cambridge Companion to Bacon*, ed. Markku Peltonen (Cambridge: Cambridge University Press, 1996), 232–59. I am grateful to Tinkler for many stimulating discussions about Bacon's views on rhetoric and natural philosophy.

47. Thomas Sprat, *The history of the Royal-Society of London for the improving of natural knowledge...* (London: T. R., 1667), 362. Two pages later Sprat writes, "It is indeed a disgrace to Reason, and honor of mankind, that every fantastical Humorist should presume to interpret the secret Ordinances of Heven."

48. An interesting exception to this tendency to avoid the theatrical analogy appears, however, in Boyle's "A Free Inquiry into the Vulgarly Received Notion of Nature," where he cautions against explaining unusual events as the result of nature's imposition on an otherwise divinely ordered world. The "ordinary and general concourse" of the laws of motion can explain both the regular course of nature and its unusual deviations, and Boyle compares the appeal to an active "nature" with the way in which bad playwrights—"for want of skill in laying the plots of their plays"—are forced to bring some deity upon the stage to "help them out." Robert Boyle, *The Works of the Honourable Robert Boyle*, 5 vols. (London: A. Miller, 1774), IV:362. Boyle prefers a rationalist poetics of divine action in the theater to a voluntarist one.

49. Given this interpretation of the spiritual function of wonder, it is not

surprising that Calvin and his followers did not want to assign a specific meaning to accidental events. Once a definitive interpretation had been found, wonder and an active sense of one's moral obligations might disappear.

50. Philip Fisher describes this process, in the Cartesian context, as the discovery that what is novel can be assimilated into a prior set of beliefs (177–78).

Bibliography

The bibliography contains items cited in the text. It is divided into sources published in the fifteenth, sixteenth and seventeenth centuries, later editions of primary sources, and selected secondary sources. Reprints or facsimiles of early sources, such as J. A. Foster's *Reprints of English Books, 1475–1700,* appear in the first section.

Works Published in the Fifteenth, Sixteenth and Seventeenth Centuries

Lamentable newes out of Monmouthshire in Wales. Contayning, the wonderfull and most fearefull accidents of the great overflowing of waters in the saide countye ... in January last 1607. London: [Edward Allde], 1607.

Lamentable newes, shewing the wonderfull deliverance of Maister Edmond Pet sayler ... Edited by Joseph Arnold Foster, *Reprints of English Books, 1475–1700.* Claremont, Calif., 1948.

More strange newes: of wonderfull accidents hapning by the late overflowings of waters, in Summerset-shire, Gloucestershire, Norfolke, and other places of England ... London: W[illiam] J[aggard], 1607.

Newes from France. A true relation of the great losses which happened by the lamentable accident of fire in the citie of Paris, the 24. day of October last past, 1621 ... London: [G. Purslowe], 1621.

Newes from Italy. Or, a prodigious and most lamentable accident lately befallen: concerning the swallowing up of the whole citty of Pleurs, belonging unto the Signiory of Venice ... London: N. O[kes], 1618.

A relation of the most lamentable burning of the cittie of Corke, in the west of Ireland, in the province of Monster, by thunder and lightning. With other most dolefull and miserable accidents, which fell out the last of May 1622 after the prodigious battell of the birds called stares, which fought strangely over and near that citie the 12. and 14. of May 1621. London: I. D., 1622.

Something written by occasion of that fatall and memorable accident in the Blacke Friers on Sonday, being the 26. of October 1623. stilo antiquo, and the 5. of November stilo novo, or Romano. [London], 1623.

A strange and miraculous accident happened in the cittie of Purmerent, on New-yeeres even last past 1599. Of a yong child which was heard to cry in the mothers wombe ... London: [E. Allde?], 1599.

A true report of all the proceedinges of Grave Mauris before the towne of Bercke... London, 1601.

A warning for all murderers. A most rare, strange, and wonderful accident, which by Gods just judgement was brought to passe, not farre from Rithin in Wales, and showne upon three most wicked persons ... London, 1620.

The wonderfull battell of starelings: fought at the citie of Corke in Ireland, the 12. and 14. of October last past. 1621 ... Edited by Joseph Arnold Foster, *Reprints of English Books, 1475–1700*. Claremont, Calif., 1948.

[Aristotle]. *The problems of Aristotle with other philosophers and physitians: wherein are contained divers questions, with their answers, touching the estate of mans body*. London: John Raworth, 1638.

Boaistuau, Pierre, and Edward Fenton. *Certain secrete wonders of nature, containing a descriptio[n] of sundry strange things, seming monstrous in our eyes and judgement, bicause we are not privie to the reasons of them*. London: Henry Bynneman, 1569.

Boethius. *Boecius de consolacione philosophie*. [Westminster: William Caxton], 1478.

Bolton, Robert. *Some generall directions for a comfortable walking with god: delivered in the lecture at Kettering in Northhamptonshire, with enlargement*. London: Felix Kyngston, 1626.

C., W. *The fatall vesper, or A true and punctuall relation of that lamentable and fearefull accident, hapning on Sunday in the afternoone being the 26. of October last, by the fall of a roome in the Black-Friers* ... London: John Haviland, 1623.

Calvin, John. *The institution of the Christian religion, written in Latine by M. John Calvine, and translated into English according to the authors last edition ... by Thomas Norton*. London: Arnold Hatfield, 1599.

Chassanion, Jean de. *The theatre of Gods judgements: or, a collection of histories out of sacred, ecclesiasticall, and prophane authours ... Translated out of French and augmented by more than three hundred examples, by Th. Beard*. London: Adam Islip, 1597.

Cooper, Thomas. *Certaine sermons wherin is contained the defense of the gospell nowe preached...* Londo[n]: Ralphe Newberry, 1580.

———. *Thesaurus linguae Romanae & Britannicae*. London, 1565.

Fielde, John. *A godly exhortation, by occasion of the late judgement of God, shewed at Parris-garden* ... London: Robert Walde-grave, 1583.

[Floyd, John.] *A word of comfort. Or A discourse concerning the late lamentable accident of the fall of a roome, at a Catholike sermon, in the Black-friars at London ... by I.R. p*. [Saint-Omer]: [English College Press], 1623.

Gataker, Thomas. *Of the nature and use of lots: a treatise historicall and theologicall; written by Thomas Gataker B. of D. The Second Edition*. London: John Haviland, 1627.

Gee, John. *The foot out of the snare with a detection of sundry late practices and impostures of the priests and Jesuits in England* ... London: H. L., 1624.

[Goad, Thomas.] *The dolefull even-song, or a true particular and impartiall narra-*

tion of that fearefull and sudden calamity, which befell the preacher Mr. Drury a Jesuite . . . London: John Haviland, 1623.

Gouge, William. *Gods three arrowes, plague, famine, sword, in three treatises.* London: George Miller, 1631.

Gribaldi, Matteo, Edward Aglionby, and Jean Calvin. *A notable and marveilous epistle of the famous doctour, Matthewe Gribalde . . . with a preface of Doctor Calvine.* London: Henry Denham [and J. Kingston?], 1570.

Hake, Edward. *Newes out of Powles Churchyarde now newly renued and amplifyed according to the accidents of the present time. 1579. and otherwise entituled, syr Nummus* . . . London: John Charlewood and Richard Jhones, 1579.

Holland, Henry. *The Christian exercise of fasting, private and publike: plainly set forth by testimonies of holy Scriptures, and also of old and late writers* . . . London: Orwin, 1596.

Hord, Richard. *Black-Fryers.* London: J. Marriot and J. Grismand, 1625.

Magini, Giovanni Antonio. *A strange and wonderfull prognostication: or rather, prenomination of those accidents which shall, or at least are likely to happen* . . . London: [E. Allde?], 1624.

Perkins, William. *A golden chaine: or, The description of theologie, containing the order of the causes of salvation and damnation* . . . [Cambridge]: John Legat, 1600.

Saxey, Samuel. *A straunge and wonderfull example of the judgement of almighty God, shewed upon two adulterous persons in London, in the parish of S. Brydes, in Fleetestreete, this thurde of Februarie. 1583* . . . London: [H. Bynneman?], 1583.

Serres, Jean de. *An historical collection, of the most memorable accidents, and tragicall massacres of France . . . Wherein we may behold the wonderfull and straunge alterations of our age. Translated out of French into English.* London: Thomas Creede, 1598.

Sprat, Thomas. *The history of the Royal-Society of London for the improving of natural knowledge*... London: T. R., 1667.

Stubbes, Phillip. *The anatomie of abuses: containing, a discoverie, or briefe summarie of such notable vices and imperfections, as now raigne in many countreyes of the world* . . . London: Richard Jones, 1583.

———. *The anatomie of abuses. Containing a description of such notable vices and enormities, as raigne in many countries of the world, but especiallie in this realme of England*... London: Richard Johnes, 1595.

———. *Two wunderfull and rare examples, of undeferred and present approaching judgement of the Lord our God the one upon a wicked and pernicious blasphemer of the name of God*... London, 1581.

Thayre, Thomas. *An excellent and best approoved treatise of the plague. Containing, the nature, signes, and accidents of the same* . . . London: [N. Okes], 1625.

Timberlake, Henry. *A discourse of the travailes of two true and strange English pilgrimes: what admirable accidents befell them in their journey to Jerusalem, Gaza, Grand Cayro, Alexandria, and other places* . . . London: [R. Bradock], 1603.

[John Wilson]. *A song, or story, for the lasting rememberance of divers famous works, which God hath done in our time.* London: R. Young, 1626.

Primary Sources

Ames, William. *The Marrow of Theology*. Translated by John D. Eusden. Durham, N.C.: Labywrinth Press, 1968.

Aquinas, Thomas. *Aquinas, Selected Philosophical Writings*. Translated by Timothy McDermott. New York: Oxford University Press, 1993.

———. *Summa contra gentiles*. Translated by Vernon J. Bourke. 3 vols. Notre Dame: University of Notre Dame Press, 1975.

———. *Summa theologiae*. Edited and translated by the Fathers of the English Dominican province. 60 vols. New York: McGraw-Hill, 1964.

Aristotle. *The Complete Works of Aristotle*. Edited by Jonathan Barnes. Princeton: Princeton University Press, 1984.

———. *Physics*. Translated by P. H. Wicksteed and F. M. Cornford. New York: G. P. Putnam and Sons, 1929.

———. *The Rhetoric and Poetics of Aristotle*. Translated by W. Rhys Roberts and Ingram Bywater. New York: McGraw Hill, 1984.

Augustine. *City of God*. Translated by Henry Bettenson. Edited by David Knowles. Baltimore: Penguin Classics, 1976.

Bacon, Francis. *Bacon's Novum Organum*. Edited by Thomas Fowler. 2d ed. Oxford: Clarendon Press, 1889.

———. *Francis Bacon: A Critical Edition of the Major Works*. Edited by Brian Vickers. Oxford: Oxford University Press, 1996.

———. *Novum Organum with Other Parts of the Great Instauration*. Edited by Peter Urbach and John Gibson. Chicago: Open Court, 1994.

———. *The Oxford Francis Bacon*. Edited by Graham Rees. Vol. VI. Oxford: Clarendon Press, 1996.

———. *The Works of Francis Bacon*. Edited by James Spedding, Robert Leslie Ellis and Douglas Denon Heath. New York: Garrett Press, 1968.

Boethius, Anicius Manlius Severinus. *Boethius's In Ciceronis Topica*. Translated by Eleonore Stump. Ithaca: Cornell University Press, 1988.

———. *The Consolation of Philosophy*. Translated by I. T. Edited by William Anderson. Carbondale, Ill.: Southern Illinois University Press, 1963.

———. *Philosophiae consolatio*. Edited by Ludovicus Bieler. Turnholti: Typographi Brepols Editores Pontificii, 1957.

Boyle, Robert. *The Works of the Honourable Robert Boyle*. 5 vols. London: A. Miller, 1744.

Calvin, John. *Institutes of the Christian Religion*. Translated by John Allen. Vol. 1. Philadelphia: Presbyterian Board of Christian Education, 1936.

———. *Institutio Christianae religionis in libros quatuor*. Edited by Baum et al. Vol. 30, *Corpus reformatorum*. Brunsvigae: A. Schewtschke et filium, 1864.

———. *Institution de la religion Chrestienne, livre premier*. Edited by Jean-Daniel Benoit. Paris: Librarie Philosophique J. Vrin, 1957.

Castiglione, Baldesar. *The Book of the Courtier*. Garden City, N.Y.: Doubleday, 1959.

Cicero. *De divinatione*. Translated by William Falconer. Cambridge, Mass.: Harvard University Press, 1974.

———. *De inventione, De optimo genere oratorum, topica*. Translated by H. M. Hubbell. Cambridge, Mass.: Harvard University Press, 1976.

[Cicero]. *Ad. C. Herennium (Rhetorica ad Herennium)*. Translated by Harry Caplan. Cambridge, Mass.: Harvard University Press, 1989.

Defoe, Daniel. *Robinson Crusoe*. Edited by Michael Shinagel. New York: W. W. Norton, 1994.

Descartes, René. *The Philosophical Writings of Descartes*. Translated by John Cottingham, Robert Stoothoff, and Dugald Murdoch. 2 vols. Cambridge: Cambridge University Press, 1985.

Farrington, Benjamin. *The Philosophy of Francis Bacon*. Chicago: University of Chicago Press, 1964.

Hansen, Bert. *Nicole Oresme and the Marvels of Nature: A Study of His De Causis Mirabilium with Critical Edition, Translation, and Commentary*. Toronto: Pontifical Institute of Mediaeval Studies, 1985.

Kant, Immanuel. *The Critique of Judgment*. Translated by James Creed Meredith. Oxford: Clarendon Press, 1989.

Lucretius. *De rerum natura*. Translated by W. H. D. Rouse. Cambridge, Mass.: Harvard University Press, 1975.

Luther, Martin. *D. Martin Luthers Werke*. 102 volumes to date. Weimar: H. Bohlau, 1883–.

———. *Works*. Edited by Jaroslav Pelikan. 55 vols. St. Louis: Concordia Publishing House, 1955–86.

Machiavelli, Niccolo. *The Prince*. Edited by Quentin Skinner and Russell Price. Cambridge: Cambridge University Press, 1995.

Magnus, Albertus. *Physica, Pars I*. Edited by Paulus Hossfeld. Aschendorff: Monasterii Westfalorum, 1987.

Matsen, Patricia P., Philip Rollinson and Marion Sousa, eds. *Readings from Classical Rhetoric*. Carbondale and Edwardsville: Southern Illinois University Press, 1990.

Paré, Ambroise. *On Monsters and Marvels*. Translated by Janis L. Pallister. Chicago: University of Chicago Press, 1982.

Plato. *Gorgias*. Translated by Walter Hamilton. New York: Penguin Books, 1960.

Platter, Thomas. *Thomas Platter's Travels in England, 1599*. Translated by Clare Williams. London, 1937.

Ramus, Peter. *The Logike of the Moste Excellent Philosopher P. Ramus, Martyr*. Translated by Roland MacIlmaine (1574). Edited by Catherine M. Dunn. Northridge, Calif.: San Fernando Valley State College, 1969.

Shakespeare, William. *The Comedy of Errors*. Edited by R. A. Foakes. Cambridge, Mass.: Harvard University Press, 1940.

———. *The Complete Works*. Edited by Stanley Wells and Gary Taylor. Oxford: Clarendon Press, 1988.

———. *Hamlet*. Edited by Horace Howard Furness. 2 vols. *A New Variorum Edition of Shakespeare*. Philadelphia: J. B. Lippincott, 1918.

———. *Hamlet*. Edited by G. R. Hibbard. New York: Oxford University Press, 1987.

———. *The Norton Shakespeare*. Edited by Stephen Greenblatt. New York: W. W. Norton, 1997.

Sidney, Philip. *An Apology for Poetry*. Edited by Forrest G. Robinson. Indianapolis: Bobbs-Merrill, 1970.

———. *The Old Arcadia*. Edited by Katherine Duncan-Jones. New York: Oxford University Press, 1994.

———. *The Countess of Pembroke's Arcadia*. Edited by Maurice Evans. New York: Penguin Books, 1977.

Spenser, Edmund. *Edmund Spenser's Poetry*. Edited by Hugh Maclean. New York: W. W. Norton, 1968.

Webster, John. *The Duchess of Malfi*. In *Five Stuart Tragedies*, edited by A. K. McIlwraith. Oxford: Oxford University Press, 1961.

———. *The White Devil*. In *Three Jacobean Tragedies*, edited by Gamini Salgado. London: Penguin Books, 1979.

Wilson, Thomas. *The Arte of Rhetorique*. Edited by G. H. Mair. Oxford: Oxford University Press, 1909.

Secondary Sources

"Kontigenz." *Poetik und Hermeneutik* 17 (1998).

Althaus, Paul. *The Theology of Martin Luther*. Translated by Robert C. Shultz. Philadelphia: Fortress Press, 1966.

Althusser, Louis. *Lenin and Philosophy and Other Essays*. Translated by Ben Brewster. New York: Monthly Review Press, 1971.

Altman, Joel B. "'Preposterous Conclusions': Eros, *Enargeia*, and the Composition of *Othello*." *Representations* 18 (1987): 129–57.

———. *The Tudor Play of Mind*. Berkeley: University of California Press, 1978.

Baker, Herschel. *The Wars of Truth*. Cambridge, Mass.: Harvard University Press, 1952.

Bal, Mieke. *Narratology*. 2d ed. Toronto: University of Toronto Press, 1997.

Barber, C. L. "Shakespearian Comedy in the Comedy of Errors." *College English* 25, no. 7 (1964): 493–97.

Barton, Ann. "Introduction to *the Comedy of Errors*." In *The Riverside Shakespeare*, edited by G. Blakemore Evans, 79–82. Boston: Houghton Mifflin, 1974.

Belfiore, Elizabeth. *Tragic Pleasures: Aristotle on Plot and Emotion*. Princeton: Princeton University Press, 1992.

Belsey, Catherine. "The Case of Hamlet's Conscience." *Studies in Philology* 76, no. 2 (1979): 127–48.

Blair, Anne. *The Theater of Nature: Jean Bodin and Renaissance Science*. Princeton: Princeton University Press, 1997.

Blumenberg, Hans. *The Legitimacy of the Modern Age*. Translated by Robert M. Wallace. Cambridge, Mass.: MIT Press, 1983.

———. *Shipwreck with Spectator: Paradigm of a Metaphor for Existence*. Cambridge: MIT Press, 1997.
Bouwsma, William J. *John Calvin: A Sixteenth-Century Portrait*. New York: Oxford University Press, 1989.
Bradley, A. C. *Shakespearean Tragedy*. London: Macmillan, 1985.
Brederkamp, Horst. *Antikensehnsucht und Maschinenglauben: Die Geschichte der Kunstkammer und die Zukunft der Kunstgeschichte*. Berlin: Klaus Wagenbach, 1993.
———. *The Lure of Antiquity and the Cult of the Machine*. Translated by Allison Brown. Princeton: Markus Wiener, 1993.
Brooks, Peter. *Reading for the Plot: Design and Intention in Narrative*. Cambridge: Harvard University Press, 1984.
Burke, Peter. *Popular Culture in Early Modern Europe*. New York: New York University Press, 1978.
Butler, Judith. "'Conscience Doth Make Subjects of Us All.'" *Yale French Studies* 88 (1995): 6–26.
Bynum, Carolyn Walker. "Presidential Address: Wonder." *American Historical Review* 102, no. 1 (1997): 1–26.
Cardwell, Kenneth William. "Francis Bacon, Inquisitor." In *Francis Bacon's Legacy of Texts*, ed. William A. Sessions, 269–89. New York: AMS Press, 1990.
Cave, Terrence. *Recognitions*. Oxford: Clarendon Press, 1988.
Céard, Jean. *La Nature et les prodiges: L'Insolite au XVIe siècle, en France*. Genève: Librarie Droz, 1977.
Chew, Samuel. "Time and Fortune." *ELH* 6, no. 2 (1939): 83–113.
Cioffari, Vincenzo. *Fortune and Fate from Democritus to St. Thomas Aquinas*. New York, 1935.
Coleridge, Samuel Taylor. *Notes and Lectures Upon Shakespeare*. Edited by H. N. Coleridge. 2 vols. London: William Pickering, 1849.
———. *Shakespearean Criticism*. 2d ed. New York: E. P. Dutton, 1960.
Crary, Jonathan. *Suspensions of Perception: Attention, Spectacle, and Modern Culture*. Boston: MIT Press, 1999.
Crewe, Jonathan V. "God or the Good Physician: The Rational Playwright in *The Comedy of Errors*." *Genre* 15, no. 1/2 (1982): 203–23.
Cunningham, J. V. *Woe or Wonder: The Emotional Effect of Shakespearean Tragedy*. Denver: University of Denver Press, 1951.
Curtius, Ernst Robert. *European Literature and the Latin Middle Ages*. Translated by Willard R. Trask. New York: Pantheon Books, 1953.
Daston, Lorraine. "Baconian Facts, Academic Civility, and the Prehistory of Objectivity." *Annals of Scholarship* 8, no. 3–4 (1991): 337–63.
———. "Marvelous Facts and Miraculous Evidence in Early Modern Europe." *Critical Inquiry* 18, no. 1 (1991): 93–124.
Daston, Lorraine, and Katharine Park. *Wonders and the Order of Nature: 1150–1750*. New York: Zone Books, 1998.
Dear, Peter. *Discipline and Experience*. Chicago: University of Chicago Press, 1995.

Derrida, Jacques. "Différance." In *Margins of Philosophy*, 1–28. Chicago: University of Chicago Press, 1982.

———. *Limited Inc.* Evanston, Ill.: Northwestern University Press, 1990.

Dickens, A. G., John Tonkin, with Kenneth Powell. *The Reformation in Historical Thought*. Cambridge: Harvard University Press, 1985.

Didi-Huberman, Georges. *Fra Angelico: Dissemblance and Figuration*. Translated by Jane Marie Todd. Chicago: University of Chicago Press, 1995.

Dolar, Mladen. "Beyond Interpellation." *Qui Parle* 6, no. 2 (1993): 75–96.

Donagan, Barbara. "Understanding Providence: The Difficulties of Sir William and Lady Waller." *Journal of Ecclesiastical History* 39, no. 3 (1988): 433–44.

Dowey, Edward A., Jr. *The Knowledge of God in Calvin's Theology*. Grand Rapids, Mich.: William B. Eerdman's Publishing, 1994.

Eamon, William. *Science and the Secrets of Nature: Books of Secrets in Medieval and Early Modern Culture*. Princeton: Princeton University Press, 1994.

Evans, Bertrand. *Shakespeare's Comedies*. Oxford: Clarendon Press, 1960.

Evans, Maurice, ed. *The Countess of Pembroke's Arcadia*. New York: Penguin Books, 1977.

Fergusson, Francis. *The Human Image in Dramatic Literature*. Gloucester, Mass.: Peter Smith, 1969.

Findlen, Paula. "Jokes of Nature and Jokes of Knowledge: The Playfulness of Scientific Discourse in Early Modern Europe." *Renaissance Quarterly* 43 (1990): 292–331.

———. *Possessing Nature: Museums, Collecting, and Scientific Culture in Early Modern Italy*. Berkeley: University of California Press, 1994.

Fisher, Philip. "The Poetics of Wonder." In *Meaning in the Visual Arts: Views from the Outside*, edited by Irving Lavin, 175–93. Princeton: Institute for Advanced Study, 1995.

Fletcher, Angus. *Allegory: The Theory of a Symbolic Mode*. Ithaca: Cornell University Press, 1964.

Foucault, Michel. *Discipline and Punish*. Translated by Alan Sheridan. New York: Vintage, 1979.

———. *Language, Counter-Memory, Practice:* Translated by Donald Bouchard and Sherry Simon. Ithaca: Cornell University Press, 1977.

———. *L'Ordre du discourse*. Paris: Edition Gallimard, 1971.

———. *The History of Sexuality*. Translated by Robert Hurley. Vol. 1. New York: Random House, 1978.

Frakes, Jerold C. *The Fate of Fortune in the Early Middle Ages: The Boethian Tradition*. New York: E. J. Brill, 1988.

Freeman, Arthur. "*The fatal vesper* and *The doleful evensong:* Claim-Jumping in 1623." *Library* 22, no. 2 (1967): 128–35.

Frye, Northrop. *Anatomy of Criticism: Four Essays*. Princeton: Princeton University Press, 1990.

Fudge, Erica. *Perceiving Animals: Humans and Beasts in Early Modern English Culture*. New York: St. Martin's Press, 2000.

Funkenstein, Amos. *Theology and the Scientific Imagination*. Princeton: Princeton University Press, 1986.

Gallagher, Catherine, and Stephen Greenblatt. *Practicing New Historicism*. Chicago: University of Chicago Press, 2000.

Gallagher, Lowell. *Medusa's Gaze: Casuistry and Conscience in the Renaissance*. Stanford: Stanford University Press, 1991.

Geneva, Ann. *Astrology and the Seventeenth Century Mind*. New York: Manchester University Press, 1995.

Ginzburg, Carlo. *Clues, Myths, and the Historical Method*. Translated by John and Anne C. Tedeschi. Baltimore: Johns Hopkins University Press, 1989.

Green, Thomas Andrew. *Verdict According to Conscience: Perspectives on the English Criminal Trial Jury 1200–1800*. Chicago: University of Chicago Press, 1985.

Greenblatt, Stephen. *Learning to Curse: Essays in Early Modern Culture*. New York: Routledge, 1992.

———. *Marvelous Possessions: The Wonder of the New World*. Chicago: University of Chicago Press, 1991.

———. *Renaissance Self-Fashioning: From More to Shakespeare*. Chicago: University of Chicago Press, 1984.

———. *Shakespearean Negotiations*. Berkeley: University of California Press, 1988.

Grennan, Eamon. "Arm and Sleeve: Nature and Custom in the Comedy of Errors." *Philological Quarterly* 59, no. 2 (1980): 150–64.

Hacking, Ian. *The Emergence of Probability*. New York: Cambridge University Press, 1975.

Harmsen, Theodorus. *John Gee's Foot out of the Snare (1624)*. Nijmegen: Cicero Press, 1992.

Hathaway, Baxter. *Marvels and Commonplaces: Renaissance Literary Criticism*. New York: Random House, 1968.

Haug, Walter. "O Fortuna." In *Fortuna*, edited by Walter Haug and Burghart Wachinger, 1–22. Tübingen: Max Niemeyer Verlag, 1995.

Haug, Walter, and Burghart Wachinger, eds. *Fortuna*. Tubingen: M. Niemeyer, 1995.

Hazlitt, William. *Characters of Shakespeare's Plays*. 2d ed. London: Taylor and Hessey, 1818.

Horkheimer, Max, and Theodor W. Adorno. *Dialectic of Enlightenment*. Translated by John Cumming. New York: Continuum, 1995.

Hunt, John. "A Thing of Nothing: The Catastrophic Body in *Hamlet*." *Shakespeare Quarterly* 39, no. 1 (1988): 27–44.

Ide, Richard S. "Shakespeare and the Pirates." *Iowa State Journal of Research* 58, no. 3 (1984): 311–18.

Jackson, James L. "'They Catch One Another's Rapiers': The Exchange of Weapons in *Hamlet*." *Shakespeare Quarterly* 41, no. 3 (1990): 281–98.

Janson, H. W. "The 'Image Made by Chance' in Renaissance Thought." In *De*

Artibus Opuscula Xl: Essays in Honor of Erwin Panofsky, edited by Millard Meiss, 254–66. New York: New York University Press, 1961.

Jardine, Lisa. "*Experientia Literata* or *Novum Organum*." In *Francis Bacon's Legacy of Texts*, edited by William A. Sessions, 47–67. New York: AMS Press, 1990.

———. *Francis Bacon: Discovery and the Art of Discourse*. Cambridge: Cambridge University Press, 1974.

Joseph, Bertram. *Conscience and the King*. London: Chatto and Windus, 1953.

Junkersfeld, Sister M. Julienne. *The Aristotelian-Thomistic Concept of Chance*. Ann Arbor: Edwards Brothers, 1945.

Keller, Evelyn Fox. *Reflections on Gender and Science*. New Haven: Yale University Press, 1985.

Kenseth, Joy, ed. *The Age of the Marvelous*. Hanover: Dartmouth University Press, 1991.

Kinneavy, James L. "*Kairos*: A Neglected Concept in Classical Rhetoric." In *Rhetoric and Praxis: The Contribution of Classical Rhetoric to Practical Reasoning*, edited by Jean Dietz Moss, 79–105. Washington: Catholic University of America Press, 1986.

Kinney, Arthur, ed. *Rogues, Vagabonds, and Sturdy Beggars: A New Gallery of Tudor and Early Stuart Rogue Literature*. Amherst: University of Massachusetts Press, 1990.

Knapp, Peggy. *Time Bound Words: Semantic and Social Economies from Chaucer's England to Shakespeare's*. New York: St. Martin's Press, 2000.

Kocher, Paul H. "Francis Bacon on the Science of Jurisprudence." *Journal of the History of Ideas* 18 (1957): 3–26.

———. *Science and Religion in Elizabethan England*. San Marino, Calif.: Huntington Library, 1953.

Kretzmann, Norman, and Eleonore Stump, eds. *The Cambridge Companion to Aquinas*. Cambridge: Cambridge University Press, 1993.

Langbein, John H. *Torture and the Law of Proof: Europe and England in the Ancien Régime*. Chicago: University of Chicago Press, 1977.

Lanier, Douglas. "'Stigmatical in Making': The Material Character of *The Comedy of Errors*." *English Literary Renaissance* 23, no. 1 (1993): 81–112.

Lezra, Jacques. *Unspeakable Subjects: The Genealogy of the Event in Early Modern Europe*. Stanford: Stanford University Press, 1997.

Long, A. A. *Hellenistic Philosophy: Stoics, Epicureans, Sceptics*. New York: Charles Scribner's Sons, 1974.

Lubac, Henri de. *Medieval Exegesis*. Translated by Mark Sebanc. Grand Rapids, Mich.: W. B. Eerdmans, 1998.

Luhmann, Niklas. *Observations on Modernity*. Translated by William Whobrey. Stanford: Stanford University Press, 1998.

Lull, Janis. "Forgetting *Hamlet*: The First Quarto and the Folio." In *The Hamlet First Published (Q1, 1603)*, edited by Thomas Clayton, 137–50. Newark: University of Delaware Press, 1992.

MacCary, W. Thomas. "The Comedy of Errors: A Different Kind of Comedy." *New Literary History* 9, no. 3 (1978): 525–36.
Mallette, Richard. "From Gyves to Graces: *Hamlet* and Free Will." *Journal of English and Germanic Philology* 93, no. 3 (1994): 336–55.
Marquard, Odo. *In Defense of the Accidental*. Translated by Robert M. Wallace. New York: Oxford University Press, 1991.
Martin, Julian. *Francis Bacon, the State, and the Reform of Natural Philosophy*. Cambridge: Cambridge University Press, 1992.
Matthews, Gareth B. "Accidental Unities." In *Language and Logos*, edited by Malcolm Schofield and Martha Craven Nussbaum. New York: Cambridge University Press, 1982.
McDonald, Russ. "Fear of Farce." In *"Bad" Shakespeare*, edited by Maurice Charney, 77–90. London: Associated University Presses, 1988.
McKeon, Michael. *The Origins of the English Novel, 1600–1740*. Baltimore: Johns Hopkins University Press, 1987.
Merchant, Carolyn. *The Death of Nature: Women, Ecology and the Scientific Revolution*. San Francisco: Harper Collins, 1980.
Metz, Christian. *The Imaginary Signifier: Psychoanalysis and the Cinema*. Translated by Celia Britton et al. Bloomington: Indiana University Press, 1977.
Meyer, Susan Suavé. "Aristotle, Teleology, and Reduction." *Philosophical Review* 101, no. 4 (1992): 791–825.
Mirollo, James V. "The Aesthetics of the Marvelous: The Wondrous Work of Art in a Wondrous World." In *The Age of the Marvelous*, edited by Joy Kenseth. Hanover: Dartmouth University Press, 1991.
Muir, Kenneth. "Comic Tradition and the European Context: The Testing of Love." In *Comedy from Shakespeare to Sheridan*, edited by A. R. Braunmuller and J. C. Bulman, 53–73. Newark: University of Delaware Press, 1986.
———, ed. *Shakespeare: The Comedies: A Collection of Critical Essays*. Englewood Cliffs, N.J.: Prentice-Hall, 1959.
Mullaney, Steven. "Strange Things, Gross Terms, Curious Customs: The Rehearsal of Cultures in the Late Renaissance." In *Representing the English Renaissance*, edited by Stephen Greenblatt, 65–92. Berkeley: University of California Press, 1988.
Mulligan, Lotte. "Puritans and English Science: A Critique of Webster." *ISIS* 71, no. 258 (1980): 456–69.
Nerlich, Michael. *Ideology of Adventure: Studies in Modern Consciousness, 1100–1750*. Minneapolis: University of Minnesota Press, 1987.
Niccoli, Ottavia. *Prophecy and People in Renaissance Italy*. Translated by Lydia G. Cochrane. Princeton: Princeton University Press, 1990.
Nietzsche, Friedrich. *On the Genealogy of Morals*. Translated by Walter Kaufman and R. J. Hollingdale. New York: Vintage Press, 1989.
Orgel, Stephen. *The Illusion of Power: Political Theater in the English Renaissance*. Berkeley: University of California Press, 1975.
Osler, Margaret J. *Divine Will and the Mechanical Philosophy: Gassendi and Des-*

cartes on Contingency and Necessity in the Created World. Cambridge: Cambridge University Press, 1994.

The Oxford English Dictionary. 2d ed. Prepared by J. A. Simpson and E. S. C. Weiner. Oxford: Clarendon Press, 1989.

Ozment, Steven. *The Age of Reform, 1250–1550: An Intellectual and Religious History of Late Medieval and Reformation Europe*. New Haven: Yale University Press, 1980.

Palmer, D. J. "The Early Comedies." In *Shakespeare: Select Bibliographical Guides*, edited by Stanley Wells, 54–73. Oxford: Oxford University Press, 1973.

Park, Katharine, and Lorraine Daston. "Unnatural Conceptions: The Study of Monsters in Sixteenth- and Seventeenth-Century France and England." *Past and Present* 92 (1981): 20–54.

Parker, Patricia. "Anagogic Metaphor: Breaking Down the Wall of Partition." In *Centre and Labyrinth: Essays in Honour of Northrop Frye*, edited by Elanor Cook et al., 38–58. Toronto: University of Toronto Press, 1983.

———. *Inescapable Romance: Studies in the Poetics of a Mode*. Princeton: Princeton University Press, 1979.

———. *Literary Fat Ladies: Rhetoric, Gender, Property*. New York: Methuen, 1987.

———. "*Othello* and *Hamlet:* Dilation, Spying, and the 'Secret Place' of Woman." *Representations*, no. 44 (1993): 60–95.

———. "Shakespeare and the Bible: *The Comedy of Errors*." *Recherches sémiotiques/Semiotic Inquiry* 13, no. 3 (1993): 47–72.

Patch, Howard R. *The Goddess Fortuna in Mediaeval Literature*. Cambridge: Harvard University Press, 1927.

Pérez-Ramos, Antonio. *Francis Bacon's Idea of Science and the Maker's Knowledge Tradition*. Oxford: Clarendon Press, 1988.

Pitkin, Hanna Fenichel. *Fortune Is a Woman: Gender and Politics in the Thought of Niccolo Machiavelli*. Chicago: University of Chicago Press, 1999.

Pollard, A. W., and G. R. Redgrave. *A Short-Title Catalogue of Books Printed in England, Scotland and Ireland, 1475–1640*. 2d ed. 3 vols. London: Bibliographical Society, 1986.

Pomian, Kryzysztof. *Collectors and Curiosities: Paris and Venice, 1500–1800* [1987]. Translated by Elizabeth Wiles-Portier. Cambridge: Polity Press, 1990.

Popkin, Richard. *The History of Scepticism from Erasmus to Descartes*. Rev. ed. Assen: Van Gorcum, 1964.

Prest, Wilfred R. *The Inns of Court under Elizabeth I and the Early Stuarts: 1590–1640*. Totowa, N.J.: Rowman and Littlefield, 1972.

Primack, Maxwell. "Outline of a Reinterpretation of Francis Bacon's Philosophy." *Journal of the History of Philosophy* 5, no. 2 (1967): 123–33.

Reichert, Klaus. *Fortuna oder die Beständigkeit des Wechsels*. Frankfurt: Suhrkamp, 1985.

Rheinberger, Hans-Jörg. *Toward a History of Epistemic Things: Synthesizing Proteins in the Test Tube*. Stanford: Stanford University Press, 1997.

Rosador, K. Tetzeli von. "Plotting the Early Comedies: 'The Comedy of Errors,'

'Love's Labour's Lost,' 'The Two Gentlemen of Verona.'" *Shakespeare Survey* 37 (1984): 13–22.

Ross, David. *Aristotle*. New York: Routledge, 1995.

Rossi, Paolo. *Francis Bacon: From Magic to Science*. Translated by Sacha Rabinovitch. London: Routledge and Kegan Paul, 1968.

Salgado, Gamini. "'Time's Deformed Hand': Sequence, Consequence, and Inconsequence in 'The Comedy of Errors.'" *Shakespeare Survey* 25 (1972): 81–91.

Salingar, Leo. *Shakespeare and the Traditions of Comedy*. Cambridge: Cambridge University Press, 1974.

Saxonhouse, Arlene W. "Review of *Fortune Is a Woman*, by Hanna Fenichel Pitkin." *Ethics* 105 (1985): 759–61.

———. *Women in the History of Political Thought: Ancient Greece to Machiavelli*. New York: Praeger, 1985.

Sayre, Francis Bowes. "Mens Rea." *Harvard Law Review* 45, no. 6 (1932): 974–1026.

Seaver, Paul. *Wallington's World: A Puritan Artisan in Seventeenth-Century London*. Stanford: Stanford University Press, 1985.

Serjeantson, R. W. "Testimony and Proof in Early-Modern England." *Studies in History and Philosophy of Science* 30, no. 2 (1999): 195–236.

Sessions, William A., ed. *Francis Bacon's Legacy of Texts*. New York: AMS Press, 1990.

Shapin, Steven, and Simon Shaffer. *Leviathan and the Airpump: Hobbes, Boyle, and the Experimental Life*. Princeton: Princeton University Press, 1985.

Shapiro, Barbara. *Probability and Certainty in Seventeenth-Century England*. Princeton: Princeton University Press, 1983.

Shelburne, Steven R. "The Nature of 'Error' in *The Comedy of Errors*." *Explorations in Renaissance Culture* 18 (1992): 137–51.

Shuger, Debora. *Habits of Thought in the English Renaissance: Religion, Politics, and the Dominant Culture*. Berkeley: University of California Press, 1990.

Sinfield, Alan. *"Hamlet's Special Providence." Shakespeare Survey*, vol. 33. New York: Cambridge University Press, 1980.

Smith, Lacey Baldwin. *Treason in Tudor England: Politics and Paranoia*. Princeton: Princeton University Press, 1986.

Solmsen, Friedrich. "Nature as Craftsman in Greek Thought." *Journal of the History of Ideas* 24, no. 4 (1963): 473–96.

Theisen, Joachim. "Fortuna Als Narratives Problem." In *Fortuna*, edited by Walter Haug, 143–91. Tübingen: Max Niemeyer Verlag, 1995.

Thomas, Keith. *Religion and the Decline of Magic*. New York: Oxford University Press, 1971.

Tinkler, John. "Bacon and History." In *The Cambridge Companion to Bacon*, edited by Markku Peltonen, 232–59. Cambridge: Cambridge University Press, 1996.

Todd, Margo. "Providence, Chance and the New Science in Early Stuart Cambridge." *Historical Journal* 29, no. 3 (1986): 697–711.

Todorov, Tzvetan. *The Fantastic: A Structural Approach to a Literary Genre*. Translated by Richard Howard. Ithaca: Cornell University Press, 1975.

Untersteiner, Mario. *The Sophists*. Translated by Kathleen Freeman. Oxford: Basil Blackwell, 1954.

Urbanas, Alban. *La Notion d'accident chez Aristote: Logique et métaphysique*. Paris: Belles Lettres, 1988.

VanderMolen, Ronald J. "Providence as Mystery, Providence as Revelation: Puritan and Anglican Modifications of John Calvin's Doctrine of Providence." *Church History* 47, no. 1 (1978): 27–47.

Warburg, Aby. *The Renewal of Pagan Antiquity*. Translated by David Britt. Los Angeles: Getty Research Institute, 1999.

Warner, William Beatty. *Chance and the Text of Experience: Freud, Nietzsche, and Shakespeare's Hamlet*. Ithaca: Cornell University Press, 1986.

Watt, Tessa. *Cheap Print and Popular Piety, 1550–1640*. Cambridge: Cambridge University Press, 1991.

Wheale, Nigel. *Writing and Society: Literacy, Print and Politics in Britain 1590–1660*. New York: Routledge, 1999.

Williams, Raymond. *Keywords: A Vocabulary of Culture and Society*. Oxford: Oxford University Press, 1976.

Wilson, Luke. "*Hamlet*, Hales V. Petit, and the Hysteresis of Action." *ELH* 60 (1993): 17–55.

Witmore, Michael. "Guarantees of the Remarkable." *Qui Parle* 6, no. 2 (1993): 1–40.

Wittkower, Rudolf. "Chance, Time and Virtue." *Journal of the Warburg Institute* 1 (1937–38): 313–21.

Index

In this index an "f" after a number indicates a separate reference on the next page, and an "ff" indicates separate references on the next two pages. A continuous discussion over two or more pages is indicated by a span of page numbers, e.g., "57–59." *Passim* is used for a cluster of references in close but not consecutive sequence.